MARKETS AND NETWORKS
Contracting in community health services

ROB FLYNN
GARETH WILLIAMS
SUSAN PICKARD

OPEN UNIVERSITY PRESS
Buckingham • Philadelphia

1H048838

Open University Press
Celtic Court
22 Ballmoor
Buckingham
MK18 1XW

and
1900 Frost Road, Suite 101
Bristol, PA 19007, USA

First published 1996

A catalogue record of this book is available from the British Library

ISBN 0 335 19456 7 (pb)   0 335 19457 5 (hb)

Library of Congress Cataloging-in-Publication Data
Flynn, R. (Robert), 1951–
    Markets and networks : contracting in community health services /
Rob Flynn, Gareth Williams, and Susan Pickard.
        p. cm.
    Includes bibliographical references and index.
    ISBN 0-335-19457-5   ISBN 0-335-19456-7 (pbk.)
    1. Community health services—Business management.   2. Contracting
out.   I. Williams, Gareth, MD.   II. Pickard, Susan.   III. Title.
RA410.5.F69   1996
362.1'0425—dc20   96–22704
                                                          CIP

Typeset by Dorwyn Ltd, Rowlands Castle, Hants
Printed in Great Britain by St Edmundsbury Press, Bury St Edmunds, Suffolk

MARKETS AND NETWORKS

Contracting in community health services

Contents

Acknowledgements

We wish to record the financial support of the Economic and Social Research Council: this book represents one of the products of a project (L114251003) funded by the ESRC through its 'Contracts and Competition' Programme. Other programme team members have been stimulating colleagues, especially, until his sad death, our colleague and friend, Kieron Walsh.

We also wish to thank the many National Health Service managers and professionals who enabled us to carry out intensive fieldwork with them over a period of two years, and to pay tribute to them not only for helping us and putting up with our questions, but also for their resilience in coping with the NHS internal market.

Our families and friends have also borne the brunt of our preoccupations, and had to endure the encroachment of our work on their lives: we thank them for their help.

We want to thank Carole Maloney for her help on the project, and our colleagues in the Department of Sociology, Institute for Social Research, and Public Health Research and Resource Centre at the University of Salford for various forms of support. In particular we wish to acknowledge Elaine Baldwin, Chris Bryant, Vic Duke, Steve Edgell, Brian Longhurst and Jennie Popay.

Introduction

During the 1980s, the welfare state in the UK and other advanced capitalist states underwent profound changes, driven by both expenditure crises and ideological critiques. The political paradigm of the New Right became dominant, entailing a radical review of the scale and scope of state intervention, especially in social policy. In the UK, as elsewhere, public spending on health care was a cause of major concern, as demand increased, demographic trends intensified claims on resources, and innovations in medical technology extended the range of possible treatments. Throughout Europe and North America, health-care systems became the target of cost-containment programmes and organizational reform.

The resulting strategy, adopted by many different countries, comprised the application, or restoration, of market principles to formerly publicly financed and publicly provided health-care systems. In the UK, because of widespread political support for the National Health Service (NHS), the Government recognized that outright privatization was not feasible, and so from 1991 introduced a massive restructuring process based on the idea of an 'internal market'. Within a universal, tax-funded system, the provision of health services was separated from purchasing, and competition between hospitals and other provider units was expected to stimulate greater cost-efficiency and improved quality. For this quasi-market to work, it was necessary to implement a complex contracting process to enable purchasers to specify needs and objectives and to negotiate and monitor services, prices and quality with various providers.

Much of the academic discussion and public debate about these changes has been focused on their impact in acute hospital-based services and also the potential inequities resulting from general practitioner (GP) fundholding. By comparison, relatively little attention has been given to a very important, but largely unacknowledged sector of health care, i.e. community health services (CHS). Briefly, CHS comprise district nursing, health visiting, and therapeutic treatment and rehabilitation, which are carried out in patients' homes, as well as preventative, screening and health-promotion work undertaken in local primary-care settings. Partly because of well-established and traditional medical dominance, the obvious urgency attached to treatment of acute conditions in hospitals, and the visibility of high technology and curative medicine, primary care, community nursing and therapeutic work receive much less recognition (and fewer resources).

Given that there is now an impetus to treat more patients in the community through expanding GP and related primary care, however, CHS have become increasingly important: reduced lengths of stay, faster throughput in and earlier discharge from hospitals, and increased demand for the 'extra-mural' management of chronic illness, disability and mental illness. There are about 60 specialized CHS Trusts in England, with a further 23 combined acute and community Trusts, and about 60 Trusts combining community services with those for mental illness and learning disabilities. In 1994–5, NHS expenditure on CHS was £2954 million, comprising 13 per cent of total revenue expenditure (NHS Executive 1996). There were 15 641 district nurses and 10 135 health visitors in England, and these community nurses and other paramedical staff carried out 122 454 000 contacts with patients in 1994–5 (Health and Personal Social Services Statistics 1995).

In addition to their growing importance in the provision of community- and domiciliary-based care, CHS are especially significant because their work necessitates considerable professional autonomy and discretion. They are located in, and exemplify, a *network* form of organization and involve continuous collaboration and coordination with many other health-service workers, statutory and voluntary agencies, patients and informal carers. These features make the application of quasi-market competition and contracts problematic, and it is indeed questioned whether the NHS internal market and commodified exchange relations may have corroded some of the essential values of trust and network structures which are claimed as integral to CHS.

This book, therefore, examines the intersection of markets and networks in CHS through a detailed analysis of qualitative evidence drawn from a recent Economic and Social Research Council project, ('Contract specification and implementation in community health services', October 1992–September 1995, project L114251003) and relates the findings to broader debates about quasi-markets and the contracting culture. The discussion is based on case studies of the process of contracting in three areas over two years which consisted of extended observation and interviewing with health authority purchasers, CHS provider Trusts, GP fundholders and GPs, and representatives of patients, carers and users. The findings are presented and compared area by area. Three case study areas within one English NHS region were initially selected because they had different organizational and strategic approaches to commissioning and contracting and because they contained a variety of different types of CHS provider. These areas were metropolitan–urban, containing deprived inner-city localities as well as more affluent suburbs. They are referred to as Areas 1, 2 and 3 (see Appendix for details of the methodology).

The main objective of the book is to present a 'policy ethnography' which gives an in-depth understanding of key actors' experiences and meanings as they designed, bargained, managed and coped with contracts for CHS. While the case studies and qualitative methods do not permit statistical generalization, we are confident that the data collected are high in validity, and (in the light of comparison with other evidence elsewhere) are broadly typical. The book reflects both the contingencies of research design and resources, as well as variations in the salience of issues in the case-study areas. The aim is to present an empirically-grounded qualitative analysis of the *process* of contracting, and to give a sociological account of practitioners' experiences. Consequently, detailed narrative accounts of the preparation and implementation of quasi-market contracts are given.

Chapter 1 outlines the theoretical and policy context surrounding the introduction of quasi-markets in CHS. Chapter 2 presents empirical material illustrating the problematic and socially constructed meanings of CHS, and discusses the local implications of alternative conceptualizations. Chapter 3 considers the ways in which purchasers and providers approached the assessment of health needs and outcomes in the contracting process. Chapter 4 focuses upon the extent to which the views of users or potential consumers were incorporated in commissioning and contracting. Chapter 5 reviews evidence about GP fundholders' paradoxical attitudes towards the purchasing of CHS. Chapter 6 contains a necessarily lengthy and detailed analysis of the contract negotiations between health authority purchasers and CHS Trusts. Chapter 7 highlights some of the strategies used by purchasers to monitor contracts and manage providers' performance and quality. Finally, Chapter 8 gives an overview of the main findings, and argues that quasi-market contracting may weaken the inherent network form and essential 'high-trust values' embedded in CHS.

1

Quasi-markets and community health services

The Introduction has noted that in common with many other capitalist industrial societies, the welfare state in the UK underwent significant transformation in the 1980s. The NHS was a keystone of the welfare state and consumed vast amounts of resources, so it inevitably featured as a candidate for reform and as a source of continuous political controversy. The Government identified a number of interlinked problems – the absence of incentives for efficiency, the lack of responsiveness to consumers and the need for more devolved responsibility – which required fundamental organizational changes. The White Paper *Working for Patients* (Department of Health, 1989a) and eventual legislation (the NHS and Community Care Act 1990) fundamentally altered the structure and functioning of the NHS, while maintaining its status as a largely tax-funded universal public service, free at the point of use. The NHS was restructured through the establishment of a so-called 'internal market', and by the introduction of a new system of contracting between different purchasers and providers of health care services (HCS).

This chapter will discuss the nature of the internal market and examine some of the main features of quasi-markets in general. It will then consider the importance of the division of functions between different purchasers and providers. The procedures for contracting will be described, and a number of important problems – in defining activity, assigning costs and specifying quality – in the contracting process for CHS will be analysed. The dominant theme of this chapter is that there are very specific attributes of CHS which cannot be straightforwardly dealt with in contracting. It will also be argued

that the complexity, professional interdependency and interagency collaboration which characterize CHS, and which are their prerequisites, are threatened
by adversarial purchasing and provider competition. More detailed evidence
and further discussion of this argument are given later in Chapters 2 and 8.
First, however, we must consider the purposes of quasi-markets and the form
of the NHS internal market.

Quasi-markets

During the 1980s, Government concern about controlling public expenditure
was linked with more deep-rooted ideological criticisms of the welfare state.
The welfare state was regarded as inefficient, as diverting resources from
productive investment, and as debilitating people's capacity for enterprise and
self-reliance. The Governments of Margaret Thatcher and successors were
determined to carry out a radical reform of the public sector, and introduced
many measures to modernize its financial and administrative workings:
managerialism became hegemonic (see Flynn 1992a; Gray and Jenkins 1993;
Pollitt 1990).

It was realized that wholesale privatization was politically infeasible, but
decisions were taken to impose some of the methods and disciplines associated
with the commercial market. There were similar developments in the fields of
health, housing, education, and personal social services, which forced the
providers of services to respond much more directly to 'consumer' demand
and the imperative of earning revenue rather than expecting (or being guaranteed) a financial allocation. The logic which drove these changes was the
axiomatic belief that markets were the most efficient means of allocating resources and of reflecting consumer preferences, and therefore market mechanisms should be applied to public services to improve their performance, to
control their budgets, and to make them more conscious of clients or users.

Although the way in which these ideas were applied in different policy fields
was varied, there was a common principle which asserted that the state should
no longer be seen as the only, or even the dominant, supplier of welfare goods
and services. Instead, it was hoped, central government would act as the finan-
cier, underwriting investments from taxation and national insurance, and
local government and other public bodies would be the 'enablers' or facilita-
tors, and only in the last resort the direct suppliers, of public services. The
objective was a mixed economy with a plurality of providers – private/for-
profit, voluntary/non-profit and public agencies – competing with each other.
The radical innovation was the separation of payment from provision, and the
injunction that welfare-state organizations would no longer monopolize the
production and delivery of public goods and services (see Le Grand 1990;
Taylor-Gooby and Lawson 1993).

The term 'quasi-market' emerged as it was acknowledged that because of the
special nature of certain welfare goods, and because of the strong political
support in the UK for some remnants of solidaristic values, a completely free
market was impractical or undesirable. Consequently, the welfare state was

reorganized to be 'almost' a market, or 'like' a market. As Le Grand (1990) observed, this entailed far-reaching changes in both the demand and the supply sides. Consumers – or rather the parents of schoolchildren, community-care clients, or health-service patients, etc. – were no longer compelled to place themselves entirely at the discretion of their immediate local state provider. Theoretically at least, consumers carried resources with them and could exercise (limited) choice as to where and by whom they were educated, cared for, or treated. In practice, there are usually third-party agents who act on their behalf in allocating their resources and selecting their provider: education authorities, local authority care managers, GPs and health authority commissioners.

The crucial differences from previous arrangements were that providers had to demonstrate that there was genuine demand for their services, some were required to negotiate formal contractual agreements with buyers, and there was the real possibility of registering consumer dissatisfaction by withdrawing or threatening to take custom elsewhere. This was believed to be a useful way of countering the tendency to producer dominance and inertia, and the alleged propensity for tax-financed bodies to increase their costs without regard to efficiency or quality. The previous regime of central plans and formulae-based budgets (even cash-limited ones) was replaced by one which attempted to reflect local citizens' preferences and needs more accurately (though resources were still centrally cash-limited), and gave clients' representatives a kind of proxy consumer power.

On the supply side, in addition to breaking up the traditional monopoly of state providers, arrangements were set up in which suppliers had to compete directly with one another for revenue, and in some cases with the for-profit sector. Following on from earlier programmes of tendering and 'contracting out' local government services, state schools had to compete locally for pupils, residential homes had to compete for clients, hospitals had to compete for patients, and so on. State-financed providers could not set themselves up as private limited companies or become profit-making, but they were given special legal status, for example as 'opted-out' or Grant-Maintained schools and self-governing hospital and community health 'Trusts'. These were encouraged to emulate organizational and management techniques common in business enterprises and there was an expectation that they would endeavour to maximize resource growth through achieving surpluses. It was also assumed that any fall in consumer demand would be directly reflected in reduced income and thus register as an indicator of inefficiency or failure to compete. What the real outcome of insolvency might be remained obscure, but in principle there was a possibility of closure for uncompetitive suppliers, and/or takeover and rationalization by others.

There have been many criticisms of the creation of quasi-markets, pointing out that they lead to various inefficiencies or inequities of their own and that they may be the precursor or prototype of complete privatization (Deakin 1993a; Cutler and Waine 1994).

Broadly sympathetic advocates have urged that quasi-markets should be evaluated according to their impact on efficiency, responsiveness, choice, equity and quality (Bartlett and Le Grand 1993). In practice, certainly in health care, the market is not competitive. In most areas, there are usually only a few large providers and very large purchasing agencies (see Bartlett and Harrison 1993; Propper 1993) and this virtual monopoly situation is not favourable for productive efficiency. In an evaluation of the impact of the NHS internal market, Le Grand (1994) could not attribute undoubted improvements in cost-efficiency to the market reforms *per se*. Further, evidence about choice and responsiveness was also mixed, with GP fundholders perceiving increased choice of hospitals for referrals but other studies indicating no increase in patient choice. One of the main improvements claimed for quasi-markets is that they give consumers much more influence over resource allocation, and thereby reduce bureaucratic and professional paternalism. For Saltman and von Otter (1992) consumer empowerment and patient choice was the central feature of planned markets and public competition. However, as we shall see, there are many obstacles to achieving this goal.

In relation to indicators of quality, while there are some signs of improvements in waiting times and reduced waiting lists for hospital treatment, there is no evidence of improvements in clinical care or outcomes which can be directly linked with quasi-market changes. Equity considerations are important where there are market incentives for providers (and GP fundholders) to be selective in choosing patients or clients. The evidence again is mixed in relation to GP fundholding, with some research showing no tendency towards 'cream-skimming' and other studies suggesting the emergence of a two-tier service (Le Grand 1994). Nonetheless, proponents of quasi-markets imply that these are interim results in a dynamic setting, and that gradually the reforms will secure the expected benefits.

More recent discussions have stressed that there are important differences in the market structure, information and degree of regulation found in education, health, housing and personal social services (Challis *et al.* 1994). Quasi-markets should therefore be regarded as differentiated and variable. However, Propper *et al.* (1994) have argued that there are common issues affecting most of these policy areas. First, there are so-called 'problems of market failure', where there is an imbalance in the information controlled by providers relative to purchasers, where it is difficult for new suppliers to enter the market and where evidence about outcomes is vague or unreliable. Second, there are problems with the system of commissioning and contracting, which will be discussed further below. There are also concerns that purchaser agencies may not have the requisite skills (or motivation) to act effectively as the agents for consumers. Finally, there are doubts about the extent of public accountability and user empowerment, a theme which will be pursued in detail in Chapter 4.

Many of these problems were anticipated by commentators before the NHS internal market was fully implemented (see, for example Harrison *et al.* 1989; Flynn 1992a, b; Paton 1992) but they have been experienced in different ways and to varying degrees. This variation in itself is not especially surprising given the massive organizational and cultural changes which quasi-markets entail. It may indeed reflect precisely the pluralism of a mixed economy of welfare. But it also reflects the uneven institutionalization of competitive relations, the

heterogeneity of the services, and the fundamental difficulties of devising, negotiating and monitoring contracts. In order to understand some of these issues,
we need to examine the purchaser–provider split in the NHS in more detail.

Purchaser and provider roles in the NHS internal market

Before 1991, the NHS in England was composed of 14 regional health authorities (RHAs) and about 190 subsidiary district health authorities (DHAs), operating in parallel with 90 local family health service authorities (FHSAs) for GP
and other primary care. Finance was allocated by central government to RHAs,
using a complex formula, and regions then allocated budgets to districts for
hospital and community services while FHSAs reimbursed GPs and met the
costs of GP drug prescribing. The DHAs were directly responsible for the service planning, management and budgets of all hospital and community units.
    One of the main assumptions of the 1989 reforms was that this structure
produced cost-inflation and resource inefficiency, and it was believed that
hospitals had little incentive to become more efficient. Central government,
seeking more stringent cost controls, endorsed the view that the NHS was
dominated by medical professionals and argued that this system was based on
'producer capture' and had to be broken up. Debates about policies and resources were thought to be rigidly constrained by thinking in terms of current
service providers' interests rather than patients' needs and preferences. Consequently, the key element of the reforms was to force producers to become
more responsive to users or consumers by separating the functions of funding
from delivering health care (for detailed accounts of the structural reorganization, see Harrison *et al.* 1990; Ham 1994a).
    The purchaser–provider split in the NHS thus involved making the suppliers
of health-care services (NHS hospitals and community health services) separate units from the purchasers (the DHAs and fundholding GPs). The districts
were to be funded according to their resident population numbers, weighted
for age, sex and morbidity, and they were required to buy services from a
variety of providers. Crucially, local hospitals and community units would no
longer be guaranteed resources by the local DHA or GP fundholders, and
instead were forced to compete for their business. Initially, not all hospitals
and community units obtained self-governing Trust status, and for a period
many remained in the anomalous position of being 'DMUs' (directly managed
units responsible to their parent DHA). This gradually changed so that by 1994
the majority (about 450) of acute hospitals, mental health and community
units had acquired Trust status.
    As experience with the internal market accumulated, and central govern-
ment's strategic concerns about regulation evolved, the number of DHAs was
reduced (through amalgamations) and from April 1995 they were effectively
merged with FHSAs forming about 90 integrated 'health commissions'. At the
same time, RHAs underwent both a numerical reduction to eight and changes
in function, becoming explicitly executive agencies (Regional Offices) of the
Department of Health (NHS Executive, Department of Health, 1994).

The establishment of fundholding for GPs was much slower to develop, largely because of widespread opposition from many doctors and criticism from their professional bodies, as well as limitations owing to practice size. Essentially, GP fundholders were allocated a budget directly by their RHA (based on existing or historical referral patterns and deducted from the district allocation), and they could use this budget to buy selected hospital inpatient services, outpatient treatments, diagnostic tests, drugs and to pay for practice administrative staff and equipment (for an extended analysis, see Glennerster *et al.* 1994). Community health services were added to the fundholding scheme in 1993 (see Chapter 5). By 1995 there were 10 410 GP fundholders in 2603 practices in England, covering 41 per cent of the population (Health and Personal Social Services Statistics 1995: 105). Services for the patients of non-fundholding GPs were the subject of much larger separate contracts drawn up by DHA purchasers.

The importance of the purchaser–provider split cannot be underestimated, because it radically altered roles and responsibilities at all levels. As Appleby (1994) noted previously, the NHS had been in effect a command economy, but even with continued central budgetary control, the NHS internal market introduced managed competition between hospitals and other providers and this completely transformed relationships between all of the interest groups and agencies. Providers were forced to consider how they could secure their income through contracts, and this necessitated business planning and marketing strategies. District health authorities' purchasing responsibilities consisted of assessing the health needs of their resident population, identifying service requirements, negotiating contracts with various providers, and monitoring the effectiveness and outcomes achieved by those providers. For all actors, this demanded a significant change in organizational and professional culture (see Appleby *et al.* 1990; Ham 1994a). According to the Audit Commission (1993: 5): 'Districts are having to make radical changes to their own objectives, cultures and working practices,' and these changes were echoed within provider units and Trusts.

The transition to a new environment was relatively slow and difficult for many of the agencies involved. The Government, prior to a general election and fearful of the political impact of disruptive changes, advised NHS purchasers and providers to implement the reforms gradually, with contracts maintaining a 'steady state' in 1991–2. In reality, this meant that existing patterns of provision were to be continued and major changes in services (or closures of large hospitals) were to be avoided, as organizations and people adapted to their new responsibilities (see Ham 1994a). Subsequently, ministers encouraged purchasers to take a more active approach towards providers, resulting in well-publicized incidents of specialty and hospital closures and mergers in many large cities and especially in London.

Such evidence as was available about purchaser managers' attitudes to their new roles suggested that they relished the opportunity to exercise more influence on providers, but also an acknowledgement that inadequate resources were still a major problem. In one study in 1991, 88 per cent of district general managers believed that the reforms would make the NHS more business-like

and this was a good thing; 55 per cent believed the market would work successfully. In a follow-up survey, while managers gave the highest priority to
obtaining equal access to services for their local population, and buying the
same amount of health care but with improved quality, the *lowest* priority was
to protect the provider units in their own district (Appleby *et al.* 1991; Appleby
et al. 1992). Concerns about the impact of such developments, together with
anxiety about the effects of GP fundholding, resulted in a pragmatic recognition that the internal market could not sustain unhindered competition but
had to be actively managed and regulated (see Ferlie *et al.* 1993; Spurgeon
1993; Ham 1994b).

Relationships between purchasers and providers take many forms, reflecting
statutory requirements, local history and immediate issues. In the internal
market, however, contracts are the main mode of, or instrument for,
interorganizational exchange. Among the very few empirical studies of NHS
contractual behaviour, a wide degree of variation has been found in
purchaser–provider relationships. In the first years of contracting, in some
areas there were both adversarial and cooperative styles (Harrison and Wistow
1992) whereas in others, 'relationships have varied between what appeared a
rather cosy and comfortable existence to political chaos and absence of
communication' (Freemantle *et al.* 1993: 538).

The Audit Commission (1993: 75) observed that some newly-formed
hospital and community Trusts were 'keen to exercise their independence
from DHAs . . . and reluctant to disclose financial information, especially cost
structures, to purchasers in general,' whereas in many areas, purchasers were
so closely linked with their main providers there was little freedom to alter
services except in marginal ways. Official guidance to DHAs seemed to vary
between exhortation to become more effective purchasers by stressing the
need for value for money as well as clinical effectiveness, to encouragement to
develop shared understandings and mutual cooperation with main providers.
Instructions on commissioning and contracting thus contained ambivalent
values, and can be interpreted as mandating assertive or adversarial purchasing
as well as collaborative and partnership approaches in contracting.

The first crucial issue is whether the purchasers (DHAs and GP fundholders)
wish, with their resources, to maintain, reduce or expand the amount of
services bought from a current provider, and make changes in the form and
quality of service delivery; or whether they will seek extra or alternative
suppliers to supplement or replace their traditional providers. District health
authorities as purchasers are largely governed by national and regional
priorities in connection with client groups and types of services to be
developed, and local purchasing plans allow only very limited scope for
specific variations on these (see Chapter 2). Annually, central guidance
virtually instructs DHAs what their priorities must be, and districts tailor these
to particular local objectives, dependent on funding, which then form
the basis for contract negotiations with providers. General practitioner
fundholders have relatively more freedom in selecting those services (and
providers) which they wish to commission using their devolved budget, and
comparatively greater flexibility in the use of that budget. Both types of

purchaser are thus assumed to have a high degree of commitment to achieving the maximum health gain and value for money through contracts.

The second issue is one of how constrained provider Trusts are to meet the purchasers' contract requirements: some Trusts may have a large dominant purchaser and little opportunity to sell services to other purchasers, for example. Conversely, certain acute specialties may have very high levels of demand from numerous potential purchasers and thus have greater bargaining power. The virtues of Trust status were based on autonomy, the ability to own and trade assets, to borrow money for capital developments, to employ their own staff, and to sell their services through contracts. All costs have to be covered, a 6 per cent return on capital is expected, and surpluses can be retained (NHS Management Executive, 1990a). In practice, Trusts have been subject to close inspection and regulation by the NHS Executive, and financial constraints (relayed through purchasers' contracts) place limits on their activity. Nonetheless, Trusts are assumed to be independent and business-like – identifying market opportunities and developing business plans – and are required to demonstrate their efforts to improve cost-efficiency and improved standards of services. Given this, they are totally dependent on revenue from contracts, and it can be assumed that they will approach the contracting process purposefully, seeking to maximize their income.

The contracting process

Contracts are formal agreements to exchange goods or services and are the essential medium for markets to operate. In the NHS internal market, contracts are 'the subject of agreement between purchaser and provider and . . . specify the nature and level of service which the provider is expected to give and the basis upon which the cost of those services will be reimbursed' (Department of Health 1989c: 7). Such contracts also comprise details of arrangements for information, for monitoring and for changes in the terms and conditions of the contract.

Only NHS contracts with private sector bodies are strictly legal commercial contracts. NHS internal market contracts are *not* legally enforceable: internal 'contracts' are not voluntary, prices are heavily regulated, and disputes are resolved administratively (there are no mechanisms for judicial determination in the case of non-compliance) (Chalkley and Malcomson 1994; Allen 1995; Jost *et al.* 1995). Nevertheless, they are the foundation for the reformed system of commissioning in the NHS quasi-market and constitute the primary device for ensuring accountability for expenditure and meeting policy goals. Payment to providers for services is channelled through the contracting process, by both GP fundholders and health authority purchasers.

There are broadly three types of contract: block, cost and volume, and cost per case.

- Block contracts enable purchasers access to a range of specified services for a fixed payment, for example, with conditions attached relating to waiting times and quality of performance. In this situation, providers bear a large risk if the numbers of patients treated exceeds expected targets and costs increase. However, it is also possible for providers to act opportunistically, reducing their costs by allowing quality to deteriorate, if there are vague or inadequate safeguards written into the contract.

- Cost-and-volume contracts permit providers to treat a certain number of patients or carry out a specified number of treatments for a predetermined price, and after reaching an agreed threshold, additional cases would be paid for at average or marginal costs. Risks are thus more evenly spread between purchasers and providers.

- Cost per case contracts were anticipated as being appropriate for highly specialized or infrequent treatments: payment depends solely on each individual case, with no guarantee by either party of the total volume of cases. Glennerster *et al.* (1994) indicate that some GP fundholders preferred the flexibility and control offered by cost per case contracts, but as Bartlett (1991) has pointed out, such contracts require sophisticated information about cases, quality and prices, resulting in very high administrative costs.

Largely due to the organizational difficulties of establishing the purchaser–provider split, early experience of contracting was dominated by the prevalence of block contracts (National Audit Office 1995). In 1993, under strong pressure by the NHS Executive, health authorities were urged to develop more sophisticated types of block contracts, stipulating minima ('floors') and maxima ('ceilings') for case-loads and more specific indicators for quality and outcomes, with the prospect of financial incentives and penalties for these targets. A departmental review of developments in contracting found that 'sophisticated block contracts' accounted for 62 per cent of all DHA contracts, with the lowest percentage (54 per cent) found in community contracts. Importantly, 'simple' block contracts comprised only 5 per cent of acute but 34 per cent of community contracts (NHS Management Executive 1994). Purchasers were instructed to ensure that no simple block contracts were negotiated for 1995–6.

This then is the broad context for the process of contracting. However, one further important dimension must be stressed – the differential impact of resourcing. With the introduction of per capita funding, some districts experienced gains or losses in their financial allocations, and this directly affected their purchasing power and their negotiating stance with providers. Revenue losers could be expected to insist on protecting existing service levels and negotiate hard on price, whereas those gaining through per capita funding were expected to be able to offer positive investments to selected providers (Audit Commission 1993).

Creating contracts

In order to create a contract, certain minimal conditions or prerequisites are necessary: the object or service to be bought must be defined, the amount to be bought and sold must be agreed, the price for the exchange must be agreed, any conditions about the transaction and about quality must be set out, and terms agreed for the parties to cancel or withdraw from the contract.

In the NHS quasi-market there are fundamental problems at each stage of this process, and this is compounded by the enormous complexity of, and variation between, specialties and procedures. We argue that, *comparatively*, acute medical and surgical specialties are *relatively* easier to define, codify and calculate for contracting purposes than those elements of health services which are more continuous and comprise 'care' rather than 'cure'. Ferlie and colleagues (1993: 69) have also suggested that 'the market-like model fits relatively discrete specialties such as elective surgery more neatly than less bounded specialties like psychiatry or oncology'. However, even within the acute sector, there are difficulties in agreeing standardized systems for coding: there are 13 000 different diseases and procedures. Consequently, 'there is not, as yet, an accepted consistent way of grouping diagnoses for treatment into useful categories for contracting' (National Audit Office 1995: 12). In community health services, the range of different nursing and other para-professional staff involved, the variety of forms of treatment and settings, and the heterogeneity of clients and conditions all combine to exacerbate these inherent difficulties. Nevertheless, purchasers and providers are required to make contracts which agree activity (the volume of service), price and quality. Each aspect of the contracting process will be considered separately.

Activity

In the acute sector, activity is conventionally defined in terms of finished consultant episodes (FCE) but in CHS, activity is usually measured by 'community contacts' (that is, visits or treatments by district nurses, health visitors, etc.). The workload of whole-time equivalent staff in previous years is thus the basis for annual negotiations about future activity. Two major problems have been observed and are common to all CHS Trusts. First, what counts as a community contact is vague and subject to variable interpretation. Second, routine coding and counting of this workload has been hampered by inadequate (or sometimes non-existent) computer information systems, and particularly by problems in collating data about individual patients seen by different professionals. Both problems make contracting negotiations and especially monitoring particularly difficult (NHS Management Executive 1993a).

In various projects to improve information systems, it was recognized that current data and recording procedures (based on patient contacts) bore little or no relationship to patient needs, the actual nature of service delivery, or outcomes achieved. Various attempts were made to improve matters, and experimental schemes were introduced to move towards an agreed basis for defining 'care objectives' and programmes of care, against which various professional activities could be counted, costed and assessed (NHS Management Executive 1993b). Both providers and purchasers have been shown to be dissatisfied with conventional information systems: 'Providers are generally in agreement that there needs to be a move away from an activity based approach to contracting for care with contacts described in a more meaningful and relevant way . . .

Purchasers focus on activity data simply because this is all that is currently available' (NHS Management Executive 1993c: 17).

This national picture was confirmed in all three of our case-study sites. The crudity and unreliability of activity statistics were frequently stressed by provider managers in interviews. Even where significant improvements in record-keeping and data analysis had been obtained, there was widely acknowledged doubt about the meaning and validity of patient contacts as the basis for activity. Providers argued that with increased patient dependency requiring more intensive community nursing, there were longer but fewer visits by district nurses, but crude 'contacts' underestimated their workload. Conversely, purchasers were equally aware that contacts were spurious indicators of activity and completely inadequate to evaluate outcomes and effectiveness. One commissioning manager noted that 'activity could be a note through the door or a four-hour counselling session with the family of a patient experiencing terminal illness'. Nevertheless, total staff–patient contacts remained the basic currency for all the contracting rounds we observed, but strenuous efforts were made to 'validate' the activity information, a task entered into with equal seriousness by both providers and purchasers.

Such information lies at the core of the contracting process – fixing the volume of services, agreeing costs and determining the baseline for monitoring – and was a source of contention in all three districts. In each site, special working groups or arrangements were set up to discuss information, and whether in 'contract monitoring' meetings or commissioning and negotiating meetings, there were frequent disagreements about activity levels. Providers requesting additional resources were regularly told they must supply more sophisticated and more robust information to justify their claims. These providers complained during meetings with purchasers and in interviews that these demands for information were often excessive, onerous and intrusive. Purchasers, by contrast, insisted that valid activity data was vital not just for the mechanics of contracting but in order to fulfil their commissioning responsibilities, and to demonstrate their own achievement of cost-effective health gain and improved outcomes. Arguments about the nature and appropriateness of activity information were prominent issues in routine service commissioning and monitoring meetings over a two-year period in each of the three sites. Activity was even more of a 'contested concept' in formal contract negotiations, as will be shown in later chapters.

Costs and prices

Costing in the NHS was identified as a major problem with the creation of the internal market. During the 1980s important changes had been made to improve the accounting and financial systems used, mainly to improve the identification of budgetary responsibility and expenditure control. With a quasi-market, however, new demands arose: purchasers needed consistent and reliable price information to compare the competitive efficiency of providers and providers were compelled to balance their budgets and make a 6 per cent return. The national policy requirements were that provider prices should be the same as actual costs, that costs should be 'full cost', and that providers must not cross-subsidize different contracts, procedures or specialties. Significantly, that same guidance noted: 'While great improvements are being made in contracting and management information, there is little doubt that the lack of valid, reliable and comparative data is the weak link in the contracting process' (NHS Management Executive 1993d: 1).

There were widespread problems in calculating and apportioning all the costs associated with every component of health service diagnostic, treatment and associated overhead costs (Mackerrel 1993). The Audit Commission (1993) found that providers' prices varied widely, that costing systems used were crude, and that prices quoted seemed unlikely to reflect accurately providers' real costs. In 1993 the NHS set up a national steering group on costing to standardize costing procedures for contracting but problems and inconsistencies in acute sector hospital costing have persisted (National Audit Office 1995). Dawson (1994) has criticized Department of Health guidance for being based on a fallacious model of markets, but also noted that incomplete and unsatisfactory information on prices is a major impediment to the emergence of a competitive market.

The calculation of costs is therefore an extremely problematic issue for all types of NHS health care. The basic problem is that there are a number of different dimensions of health care which have different types of cost information. Five key dimensions have been identified: clients (who is being cared for); care input (who is caring/treating); settings (where the care is given); condition (patients' clinical condition); and activity (type of care or procedure used). Studies have shown that there is much variation in the availability of data to cost these dimensions. In one study, the only dimension for which adequate cost data were available in non-acute services was 'care input', that is staff groups involved (NHS Management Executive 1993e).

In addition to these technical and methodological difficulties, there are also the consequences of market incentives. Providers may be anxious not to reveal too much about their own internal costs to purchasers, for fear of disadvantaging themselves in negotiations. They may not wish to disclose too much information about prices if this worsens their position relative to competing suppliers. The NHS Management Executive were alert to this and enjoined providers to share cost information with purchasers, since the latter had to be able to determine whether providers had improved quality and value for money: 'It is too simple to classify everything as "Commercial, in confidence" and we need to remember we are all part of one National Health Service' (NHS Management Executive 1993d: para 8). It is far from clear whether this injunction can be effective in a competitive quasi-market, and it is uncertain how costing can be resolved through annual contract negotiations.

In our case studies of CHS contracting, these general issues were recognized by both providers and purchasers as important constraints. If average specialty costs were hard to determine in hospitals, there were even more problems in aggregating the different types of work of district nurses, health visitors and community-based therapists, made more complicated by varied client groups, conditions and settings. Costs had largely been worked out on the basis of current staff establishments and historic patterns of workload, then adjusted for inflation and efficiency savings, for both DHA and GP fundholder purchasers. From April 1993, fundholders could buy community nursing directly but only on the basis of fixed-price non-attributable contracts (that is, those unrelated to individual patients).

District health authorities adopted very similar positions regarding local CHS Trust costs, with variations in stance reflecting the severity of financial problems caused by per capita funding reductions. In Area 1 (see Appendix), the purchaser in 1993–4 did not appear to attach much importance to the provider's costs as such, even though they disagreed about the funding needed to finance the provider's 'service pressures'. In Area 2 there was a strategic commitment by the purchaser to divert resources away from acute hospital service into CHS, but because of funding reductions and opposition to proposed hospital rationalizations, this transfer did not materialize. There was a constant vigilance by the purchaser about *all* providers' costs but there was no special significance attached to their local CHS Trust's costs. In Area 3 (an area with a very high ratio of fundholding GPs) the health authority did not seem particularly anxious about the community Trust costs, but the GP fundholders were. The DHA emphasized that quality issues, and changing services to meet their priority needs, were more important than prices.

From direct interviewing, it appeared that GP fundholders *were* concerned about the price of community services, and many expressed dissatisfaction about management costs for various services. They were aware of comparative cost information about different providers, and on occasion used this in bargaining. However, the majority stressed that their decision as to where to place contracts was largely influenced by their perception of the quality of service, their confidence in the professionalism of the staff, and the importance of maintaining local networks (see Chapter 5).

The DHA purchasers in interviews all emphasized that their decisions on contracts never considered cost by itself as a primary or dominant objective. Rather, the principal concerns seemed to be to maintain or increase total activity with minimal resource growth but *without* reducing quality. Overall, purchasers argued that price alone was not a crucial factor, and claimed that they were mainly seeking changes in services and linking these to their priorities and quality targets.

Quality

The other crucial dimension of any contract consists of the quality or standard of service desired by the purchaser, and the extent to which this is achieved by the provider. Basically, there are two elements to NHS contracting for quality: one consists of the specification of services required, and the other comprises the impact of services on patient care, or effectiveness. In both cases, there are conceptual and technical problems (of measurement). Further, because 'quality' necessarily entails evaluation of professionals' performance and standards, there is likely to be latent tension or even conflict about how contractual aspects of quality are managed, as Chapter 7 shows.

The NHS internal market intensified previously emerging concerns about improving service effectiveness and quality, through quality assurance, performance indicators and medical audit. All public sector services had been encouraged to emulate private commercial concerns about consumer responsiveness and standard-setting (Pollitt 1990; Audit Commission 1993). The NHS was urged to adopt methods of 'quality management' used in business to improve customer satisfaction and develop good practice in order to meet needs and maintain cost-effectiveness (Øvretveit 1992).

Broadly, two interrelated aspects have to be dealt with: one involves designing quality into contracts by making service specifications very explicit; the other is assessing the effects of treatments on patients. Again, there are considerable difficulties in doing this systematically. Kerrison (1993) has observed that quality is multidimensional and there are disagreements about the nature and legitimacy of the yardsticks used by purchasers and providers, and there are major problems in monitoring whether standards have been achieved. The measurement of health status, and the demonstration that health care, treatment or advice has resulted in identifiable and beneficial changes, is methodologically complex (Fitzpatrick 1994; Long 1994). Numerous factors influence people's health, so the measurement of outcomes linked to specific types of intervention is highly problematic.

Nevertheless, improved quality and effectiveness have become important policy goals and have been built into successive targets (for example the *Patient's Charter* and *Health of the Nation* objectives) and guidance on contracting for health authorities (NHS Executive 1995). Most of this guidance and advice concerns acute hospital services, but even in this sector, there was initially inconsistency and variability in the way in which quality was approached, and vagueness in the methods and criteria for monitoring (Maheswaren and Appleby 1992). In CHS, there has been relatively less debate about quality and very little development of procedures to assess outcomes and quality. The Audit Commission (1992: 26) commented:

> 'Clinical audit', 'management audit', 'user surveys', 'setting and monitoring standards' and 'measuring outcomes' are all now relatively familiar concepts. But they remain rare activities in the day-to-day running of community units. Few districts or provider-units have an explicit strategy that explains how quality is to be gauged or assured.

Other studies have also indicated that evaluation of the effectiveness of community nursing has been slow to develop, and that although purchasers regard quality assurance as important, the targets set varied widely in scope and detail (Lightfoot *et al.* 1992).

We argue that there are inherent problems with measuring quality in community services and that these problems cannot be solved through competitive contracting. Some of the work of district nurses may be more amenable to clinical description and evaluation than aspects of health visiting, for example, especially since the latter has more preventative and surveillance functions whose outcomes are hard to identify (Dingwall *et al.* 1988) (see also Chapter 3). Lightfoot *et al.* (1992) noted that there is a lack of agreement about what constitutes a health outcome in many types of community nursing, and that purchasers, providers and service users have different perceptions of needs and outcomes.

In the case of both district nursing and health visiting, the unresolved problem is that of demonstrating therapeutic effects, i.e. showing that measured improvements in a patient's condition or well-being have been brought about by their actions. For some of the other therapies (occupational, speech and physiotherapy), it may be relatively easier to show how much effect treatment has had, but at the boundary of health and social care, there is an important degree of uncertainty. Knapp *et al.* (1994) have argued that there are very important information imperfections in markets for services with outcomes which are uncertain, technically complex, infrequently produced, of long gestation and embodied in the characteristics of the users themselves. They also point out that these features describe virtually all social care services and that 'most social care services do not lend themselves to unambiguous and readily monitored quality standards' (Knapp *et al.* 1994: 145).

In this situation, as Propper (1993) has shown, purchasers faced with doubts about quality compliance in the contract can either attempt to specify in great detail, in advance, all the measurable dimensions of quality (but this increases the administrative burden of specification and monitoring), or they may rely upon known and trusted suppliers and/or agree upon common standards (but this may result in a lack of competition). Where it is hard to define and observe quality, Propper argues, purchasers and providers make contracts which stress inputs or processes rather than outputs or outcomes.

This indeed is what was found in our three case-study districts. Contracts either had quality specifications built into the main body of the contract document, or attached to them as separate annexes. There were, however, important differences in approach, with two DHAs acknowledging the complexity of CHS and the need for a collaborative and evolutionary approach, and the third pursuing a more bureaucratic and prescriptive approach. The latter, in Area 2, professed a desire to work collaboratively, but contract negotiators reported dissatisfaction with the Trust's apparent reluctance to devise detailed specifications. Thus, in Area 2, the purchaser quality manager acknowledged that monitoring quality was difficult and that systems had been developed in an ad hoc way:

> 'What needs to be done is to develop an understanding of what is done by providers. It's a bit like Total Quality Management, applying it to the complete process. But personal knowledge and goodwill are important, so we must start from the bottom up and make sure that quality is relevant [to providers].'

However, during contract negotiations it emerged that the DHA representatives were unconvinced that the Trust had made sufficient commitment to introduce a quality management system, and insisted on obtaining more highly formalized service and quality specifications.

Providers were very aware of the significance of quality issues and saw them as crucial to strengthening their claim for resources from their main purchasers and enhancing their marketability to prospective GP fundholders. In Area 3 for example, the clinical director for CHS had adopted a 'niche marketing' strategy to sell specialized services on the basis of their better quality as compared to other neighbouring providers. The contracts manager for this Trust endorsed this, noting that:

> 'Unless we're able to convince purchasers that clinically we're better than some of our neighbouring providers then those services . . . they're just seen as a constant . . . If they're not bad then they're all the same . . . We've certainly got to inform purchasers about the quality of the work that we are doing.'

While this was apparently straightforward for some services – palliative care in this case – others were more problematic. Indeed the head of community nursing in Area 3 acknowledged that:

> 'It is difficult to demonstrate quality in community nursing. This concerns me greatly. We think we provide a high quality service and are quite advanced and innovative . . . [but] this is a major task, demonstrating outcomes . . . [and] we have got to get to grips with this.'

Quality was thus of great concern to purchasers and providers alike. For purchasers, the principal objective was to ensure that resources are efficiently allocated to effective treatments and that strategic goals for improvements in health are secured. For providers, quality was both a feature of professional claims and Trust business marketing. In contract negotiations, therefore, quality issues were seen as important but, acknowledging the immense difficulties of specifying desired outcomes, intermediate proxies and process indicators were often preferred.

Adversarial and relational contracting

It is evident from the previous sections that in three important dimensions of the contracting process – specifying the amount to be purchased, fixing a price for the services and evaluating the quality provided – there are fundamental problems for community health services. Some of these problems are direct reflections of the intrinsic properties of CHS themselves, but some reflect the tension within the NHS between different forms of market competition and styles of contracting. From the inception of the internal market there has been a debate about how 'competitive' a market it could be, and how the contracting system could impose the dominance of purchasers. One approach stresses the importance of health commissions avoiding producer capture and instead forcing providers to compete, by drawing up stringent contractual conditions and ultimately threatening cancellation. Another approach recognizes that the NHS quasi-market is special and that medical services require a cooperative and collaborative relationship between the various agencies involved. Much of the argument about this derives from prior assumptions about how markets operate, and about what conditions are necessary to reduce opportunistic behaviour.

We therefore need to have some understanding of those key assumptions, and most importantly, an awareness of recent debates about contracting which have been dominated by the 'new institutional economics' of Williamson (1983, 1985). Williamson argued that any contractual activity can be explained in terms of economies in transaction costs – where transaction costs include *all* the costs of designing, measuring and managing the terms and conditions of exchanges between buyers and sellers. He argued that contrary to neoclassical economic theory of competitive bargaining and markets, enterprises may find it more efficient to produce and secure their materials and resources internally rather than seek to buy them from external suppliers. Contracts between organizations, according to Williamson (1983) will be attractive to the extent to which: the good or service is amenable to unambiguous written specification; joint gains from collective action are potentially available; implementation does not create costly haggling; monitoring agreements is not costly; and penalties for non-compliance can be enforced at low cost. Because people cannot have complete awareness of relevant information and because there is uncertainty about future changes there are fundamental difficulties in writing comprehensive contracts which embrace all foreseeable circumstances to regulate the exchange. Given such constraints of bounded rationality and uncertainty, complex contingent claims contracts are costly to write, implement and enforce. Organizations may thus find it more efficient to avoid this market approach to contracting and instead prefer hierarchical coordination and vertical integration.

There is a large critical literature questioning the validity of Williamson's model, particularly pointing out that many modern organizations and companies do not fit the simple dichotomy of market or hierarchy (Perrow 1981; Turk 1983; Frances *et al.* 1991). Williamson has acknowledged complex variations in organizational form and recognizes the existence of 'hybrid' modes of economic governance including the possibility of quasi-market relations (Williamson and Ouchi 1983; Williamson 1991). However, he stresses that transaction costs remain crucial determinants of the structure of exchange relationships and that this structure will be negotiated through 'private ordering' rather than through legalistic contracting (Williamson 1985).

Many other writers have shown that modern commercial and industrial companies do not engage in mutually destructive or ruthlessly competitive behaviour, but instead evolve different strategies for cooperation based on interdependence. Bradach and Eccles (1991) argued that industrial contracting is influenced by *mixtures* of price, authority and trust. Dense ties develop so that resources and knowledge are pooled and there is reciprocity between firms which are connected through alliances or networks. Powell (1991) also emphasized that if the items being exchanged between buyers and sellers are hard to measure, and/or there are repeated and long-term relations between parties, then conventional neoclassical ideas about bargaining and contracting are inappropriate. In this situation, companies create 'an intricate latticework of collaborative ventures with other firms, most of whom are ostensible competitors' (Powell 1991: 268). Network relationships formed on the basis of cooperation, obligation and trust are said to give rise to 'relational' contracts (Dore 1983; Reve 1990; Bradach and Eccles 1991).

'Hard' contracting is assumed to be characteristic of adversarial and self-interested competitive bargaining, whereas 'soft' – or relational – contracting arises from a situation of mutual benefit and an identity of interests (Williamson and Ouchi 1983). Ouchi (1991) argued that such hard contracting may be efficient where performance is straightforward and parties have common goals, and bureaucracy may be efficient if performance is ambiguous and there is little agreement about goals. However, argued Ouchi, another type of system is possible – the 'clan' system – which has advantages over both markets and bureaucracy. In a clan system, reciprocal exchanges can take place within a set of shared objectives and values: members of the clan are interdependent and obligated to others. If organizations cannot specify bureaucratic rules to cover all situations or market prices are difficult or impossible to determine, then a clan system may be the most efficient means of obtaining cooperation and coordination. These conditions apply especially among technologically advanced industries and professionalized occupations which depend on teamwork, where there are high levels of innovation, and where individual performance is ambiguous. Evidence from various studies of industrial marketing and interorganizational purchasing behaviour have also indicated that networks based on trust and reputation are increasingly significant, especially for entrepreneurial firms (Cunningham and Culligan 1990; Thorelli 1990; Larson 1992). Markets may actually be composed of networks, and there may be competition, but they do not necessarily depend on aggressive bargaining and rarely invoke the machinery of formal contracts to regulate exchange.

Conclusions

Thus several important observations must be made in relation to the NHS quasi-market. First, it is obvious that virtually none of the conditions relevant to the virtues of contracting as set out by Williamson above apply to NHS contracts: service specification is extremely problematic; implementation will entail 'haggling', since that is what follows from the need for a managed market; monitoring is complex and administratively costly; and penalties for non-compliance carry high administrative and political costs. Under these conditions there are economic efficiency grounds for favouring 'hierarchy' rather than 'market' (see Bartlett 1991).

Second, however, the NHS is a *quasi*-market and 'soft' or *relational* contracting may thus be inevitable, especially because so many of its activities involve technologically advanced and professionalized services requiring teamwork. Relational contracting and relational markets are more accurate concepts for analysing the situation where there are not many buyers and sellers, where their interaction is long term, and where there is a strong interest in reputation and quality (Ranade 1992, 1994; Maynard 1993; Ferlie 1994).

Third, it was argued earlier that CHS activity, costs and quality cannot be easily measured and translated into contractual form. Perhaps more importantly, CHS by definition exhibit many of the attributes which characterize *network* structures and 'clan' forms of organization, as we will see in Chapter 2.

Community nurses and therapists work in tandem with hospital-based health service professionals and GP-based primary health care teams, and also link up with local authority social services and voluntary agency workers. Community health services thus depend upon interagency collaboration and interprofessional cooperation. Networks, partnership and trust thus appear to be central to their operation, and so relational rather than adversarial contracting seems the appropriate mode of exchange between purchasers and providers.

What remains unclear is how the quasi-market in CHS actually functions, and how local managers and professionals in purchaser and provider agencies interpret their role in the managed market. There are contradictory rhetorics in the Government's guidance about the internal market; for example, the Department of Health has strongly advocated 'health alliances' among purchasers and providers and other agencies to maximize health gain, but simultaneously insisted on the need for purchasers to demand greater efficiency and value for money from providers (NHS Management Executive 1993d). Various commentators have observed the contradiction between strategic statements of objectives and priorities favouring collaboration, and a contracting system premissed on principles of competition. The attempt to resolve this apparent paradox has been to stress the merits of 'contestability' rather than competition (Robinson 1993; Ham 1994a). This entails the recognition that there need not be 'real' competition (with inefficient providers forced into insolvency) but rather that there should be the constant *threat* or possibility of this happening, in order to promote greater efficiency. Thus contestability means that purchasers should be able to threaten incumbent suppliers with moving contracts to alternative sources.

The Department of Health (NHS Executive 1994: 1), reviewing the degree of regulation required to manage the market, asserted that:

> We need constructive co-operation between different parts of the NHS as well as the beneficial impact of competition. Improving health care is not a question of choosing one or the other. We have to find the appropriate balance between the two.

We shall see that the degree of contestability within CHS is extremely limited and that, in practice, the balance between competition and collaboration is difficult to achieve when purchasers veer between 'hard' and 'soft' contracting, and when the contracting process exposes the limits of (and often tests) the trust essential for effective networks.

2

Conceptualizing

community health

services

The CHS represent a mixture of forms and types of provision with few obvious links between them (Ottewill and Wall 1990). Although difficult to define, they nevertheless represent one of the three arms of the NHS, alongside general practice and hospital services. The easiest way to define CHS is by saying that they are those formal health services which are not provided by GPs or in hospitals. Any introduction to the CHS contains some kind of list, and these may vary (ACHCEW 1994). However, most lists include chiropody, health visiting, family planning, school health, district nursing, community midwifery, immunization and vaccination, health education and promotion, home nursing aids, speech therapy and community dentistry.

Some community services may be provided by hospital-based professionals in people's homes. There are increasing numbers of specialist nurses, for example, who work on this outreach basis, such as stoma care and diabetic liaison nurses. Others will be provided in health centres, clinics or community hospitals, located within 'the community' close to where people live, or as part of hospital-at-home schemes. Health visitors, community midwives and district nurses are the most obvious examples of professionals providing this care. In a sense, CHS are no more or less than services described in those terms for the purposes of management. Most of what takes place within CHS can be grouped in four categories of professionals: nurses, doctors, dentists and professions allied to medicine. When we think of CHS in terms of what sort of care or intervention they provide, the particular expertise of CHS workers lies in the areas of health maintenance and health promotion, disease prevention (including monitoring and referral, rehabilitation and aftercare), and counselling and pastoral care.

In spite of the central place of these kinds of activities within any health-care system, community services have been, and continue to be, the 'poor relation' in NHS expenditure and management (Audit Commission 1992a), as we indicated in the Introduction. Although proportional expenditure on CHS has increased, they remain the poor relation in the sense that occupations within CHS are, for the most part, groups of occupations with relatively little power, and with low status and remuneration. This situation may be a reflection of the fragmented and heterogeneous nature of CHS and the shifting boundaries of the work undertaken by CHS professionals. However, it is probably also an effect of two characteristics of CHS workers: they are predominantly women and they are not doctors. Moreover, of the three sectors of the NHS – hospital, general practice and community services – it is only within CHS that the majority of the doctors who are employed are women (Department of Health 1990).

Although expenditure on CHS represents a relatively small proportion of total expenditure, these services are of large and growing significance in a health service increasingly orientated to non-hospital-based care. It has been argued that the closing years of the twentieth century are both 'the worst of times and the best of times' for CHS (O'Keefe *et al*. 1992: 1). On the one hand, policy and legislative change in health and social care, in response to demographic and epidemiological transitions, is putting these services more and more at the centre of health-service developments. On the other hand, the health-service reforms have added tensions and uncertainties to the already difficult job of health care.

The argument presented here is that the features that make community services what they are: their closeness to the lay sector of informal care, their locality orientation, and the diffuse, non-acute health needs which form a large part of the their workload, make CHS difficult to define and measure with the kind of precision necessary for the setting of formal contracts between purchasers and providers. Moreover, in contrast to many forms of acute provision within hospitals, CHS deal with the less clearly defined forms of ill health for which people require help and support in their own homes – health problems which lie on the confused and shifting boundary between health and social or community care. Services such as learning disabilities, for example, are often jointly managed between CHS and local authority social services departments. Putting these two features together, we might hypothesize that different CHS would be able to define their activities with varying degrees of precision. Chiropody might pose fewer problems for the contract specification process than district nursing, and we might expect physiotherapy to be more easily itemized and enumerated than, say, health visiting.

This chapter presents findings illustrating in some detail the problem posed by CHS for both purchasers and providers. It sets the scene for the treatment of more specific aspects of the process of contract specification and implementation which follow. However, it is important in its own right as an illustrative case of the difficulties involved in defining what particular health services are supposed to be about at a time of more general political and professional uncertainty about the organization and future of the NHS. This chapter is a detailed examination of the ways in which the problem of CHS was understood, and how it changed over the fieldwork period. The focus is the way in which CHS are defined, and the difficulties and conflicts that were encountered in doing so. The analysis is based on findings from observations of, and interviews with, members of health authorities and trusts, between 1992 and 1995, with particular attention being focused on the two contracting rounds of 1993–4 and 1994–5. We also draw upon our analysis of documentary material. The material is used to explore the process whereby the indeterminacies of CHS are defined and handled by different actors in purchaser and provider organizations and in both primary and secondary care. As will become clear, CHS have varying salience and importance for different actors and parties involved.

The analysis focuses on two crucial issues: (1) the extent to which CHS are seen to be intrinsically difficult to measure and fundamentally different from acute hospital services in this regard; and (2) the difficulties both within and between purchaser and provider organizations in applying the contents of business and purchasing plans in the harsh world of negotiating and monitoring contracts.

Defining community health services in practice

While CHS were central to the concerns of those managing the provision of them, they were not uppermost in the minds of many of the purchasers we interviewed over the fieldwork period. Also, they were always at risk of being driven to the margins by what were seen to be more pressing financial concerns. However, from very early on in our investigation, it became clear that the extent to which community health services were a problem, and for whom, was defined differently by the various actors involved.

In 1992, all the community units in the areas (see Appendix) were still directly managed, and much of the discussion among providers at that time revolved around strategies for moving to Trust status. As with so many developments, the form of CHS provision was dependent to some extent on changing policy priorities decided elsewhere. As one contracts manager for an incipient CHS Trust argued, his organization was '. . . working within broad conditions handed down from above – from regional and national levels'. Moreover, staff were already aware of a likely merger of the RHA with a smaller, more dynamic neighbouring RHA, and impending mergers of local DHAs. In these early stages of the new market, purchasers were preoccupied with dealing with the more expensive acute hospital services, and GPs were preoccupied with fundholding, whether they were advocating or resisting it.

Area 1

The DHA started out with a very clear model of purchasing which focused less on specific services and more on broader strategic issues of 'health gain'. While the chief executive (throughout the study period) was aware of the detail of organizational complexity, he and his staff attempted to keep clearly in mind the relationship between needs, resources and outcomes. To that extent, therefore, there was little discussion about the definition of CHS and more about how a variety of services, whether in the acute sector, community, or local authority social services could contribute to improvements in the health of the population. In an early discussion, the chief executive indicated that resources existed in the informal 'non-contract' sector in individuals, families and communities, and in the formal 'contract' sector at primary, secondary and tertiary levels. 'Community health services,' he argued, 'could be any of these up to the tertiary level.' He acknowledged, however, that in reality contracting for CHS is messy and there is no conceptual blueprint.

Similar views were held by the general manager of the community services unit. 'Contracting in CHS is at an early stage,' she said, 'and is difficult.' However, while the purchasers' thinking was primarily around the abstract model of linking needs to resources to outcomes, the DMU saw the advent of contracting as a 'vehicle for change', but that in CHS the lack of an adequate information base made planning difficult. In particular, it was difficult for them to identify the activity and workloads of district nurses and health visitors. In its application for Trust status, this definition of community activity was particularly important in resisting the competing 'outreach' models promulgated by the acute sector. In early 1993, the Business and Contracts Manager for the DMU said that they did not see themselves as competing with other community units in other districts, but with the acute sector in their own district.

Although the provider at this time was much more focused on the details of specific services than was the purchaser, they too recognized that CHS would have to become much more 'outcome-oriented'. However, this is difficult because 'CHS are inadequately measurable' (provider business and contracts manager), but with the increase in GP fundholding, the local nature of CHS would be increasingly important. The definition of CHS was also important to the provider in their relationship with a purchaser having such a clear 'health-gain' focus, and little concern about the formal organizational divisions between services. In the period prior to the DMU becoming a Trust, there were considerable problems of information for the provider which put them at a distinct disadvantage in their dealings with the purchasers. 'We are having difficulty with information' was a continual refrain from the providers in early 1993, and the purchasers were always having to say: 'You need to give us more data.'

The community unit became much more assertive in defining its identity after it had been given Trust status in 1993. At this time too, the purchasers were in a state of considerable uncertainty owing to negotiations over the merger of two DHAs and two family health service authorities into a single commission, with all the attendant anxieties about jobs and careers that affected the personnel at that time. The contracts manager of the new Trust told us with regard to service specifications that the Trust 'were not happy with the process of negotiation with the purchaser. They [the purchasers] wanted more information on 14 to 15 services in terms of activity and outcomes. But they [the purchasers] just accept what we tell them but don't come up with ideas and suggestions'.

The problem of defining what CHS were was therefore partly a product of lack of information and partly to do with the different levels at which purchasers and providers were interested in the issue. Although the contract was a block contract (see p. 11–12), as far as the purchaser contracts manager was concerned, it would not have been possible to have any other form, because of the dearth of information: 'We have a very good system in hospitals where they can measure FCEs, admissions, discharges, but there is no comparable system in community. The need wasn't there. Now it is.' The purchaser had no desire to interfere in the 'operational matters' of the Trust. The contracts manager saw the purchaser role as being to indicate in broad terms the kind of service and outcomes they wanted and say: 'How would you describe your business? What is the meaningful measure in your terms? Have you got the information? If you haven't got it, how can you develop it?'

There was a further way in which the CHS were difficult to define in contract terms. The purchaser had five years' data from the acute sector, and this meant that they were able to 'go to five or six different suppliers'. But '. . . it's not really appropriate to do it in a community environment . . . As a general principle it has to be community-based. So it's a bit like a "Marks and Sparks" model working with a preferred provider . . . It's a joint commissioning collaboration, but keeping an element of competition available if needs be.'

Throughout discussions with the purchasers during 1993 and 1994, there was a model of collaboration with the local community service, but with competition 'at the edges', and an emphasis on moving towards developing the 'needs–resources–outcomes' model while also developing 'a much sharper contract'. To this end, they were looking at particular areas of service and breaking them down into 'disciplines' and then within that looking at where services were being provided. From the purchaser's point of view, most CHS work seemed to be based on historical patterns that bore little relationship to the model they wanted to develop, and because of the lack of clear boundaries about who was doing what for whom, there was little usable information. Even measuring activity was something that seemed ambitious in 1993 when it was not clear what services were in place.

Within the purchaser, however, the emphasis varied between different sections of the organization. While the contracts manager emphasized the need for sharper contracting, the public health consultant leading on health needs assessment said that talking about CHS set up a 'false boundary' and would militate against a needs-led service. She argued that this emphasis on needs and outcomes was something that the provider found very difficult to deal with. Nonetheless, compared to acute sector Trusts, '. . . the management are much more open to meeting needs, much less medically and professionally dominant'. The needs–outcomes model is discussed in more detail in Chapter 3.

Meetings of purchaser and provider representatives in 1993 emphasized both the need for better information, and also according to the purchaser chief executive the necessity for 'joint work between agencies to develop a *strategy* based on needs'. The problem of information about what CHS were doing led the purchaser chief executive to argue that it's 'souring our relationship, and has gone on far too long'. The provider, however, was unsure about which information was a provider responsibility, and complained that they simply could not deliver the information the purchaser was asking for. This perception led to a great deal of anxiety particularly in the provider, and a consequent need to try and get away from business-orientated discussions about information in order to encourage, according to the purchaser contracting officer, 'openness on both sides' and 'a degree of ownership on both sides on what is being delivered'.

For the purchaser, therefore, the problem of information about what CHS actually are and do was very far-reaching. According to a public health consultant:

> 'We have no way of knowing what is going on in the community. When they refer to health visitor contacts, for example, that may involve talking to the parents of the child about a whole range of things, about family planning, about safety, about lifestyle, about all kinds of things, we have no idea.'

However, they were insistent that within the model of needs–resources–outcomes, information systems were less important than the development of constructive relationships based on a shared understanding of health needs involving collaboration between purchasers, providers, local authorities and voluntary organizations.

During 1993, the provider seemed to be very much on the defensive in discussions over what they did and how they could define and measure it. During negotiations in early 1994 over the 1994–5 contract, the discussion became much more dominated by money, and this put the problem of the lack of information into sharp focus. The following exchange between the purchaser and provider directors of contracting illustrates the difficulties involved in an information-scarce environment:

> *Purchaser director of contracting:* We've got to look at 'overheating' and 'underheating', and diversify resources from one to another – that means over- and under-activity.
> *Provider director of contracting:* It is not always possible to offset, say, district nursing versus chiropody. We've still got difficulties because of the particular arrangements we have.

The contract was eventually signed with the recognition that information about CHS activity would have to be improved over the course of the next year. The provider was quite sure that their activity was increasing in some services, and it would have benefited them to have moved to some kind of cost-and-volume contract (see p. 12) on those, but with the information so unreliable, and the 'contract currency' of counting contacts so contentious, they decided to stick with what they had. The provider sensed that there were differences within the purchaser management team and that they were unwilling to make tough decisions about investment and disinvestment based on the information the provider had collected.

As the provider became more confident during 1994 and 1995 about their own information base, so they were more prepared to challenge the purchaser over patterns of investment and disinvestment. A number of uncomfortable meetings of the joint Service Commissioning Forum took place in which the purchaser was pressed to explain and justify apparent anomalies in monies relating to investment and disinvestment, particularly relating to a health-improvement programme. The provider had become suspicious that the purchaser was not in fact as committed to CHS developments as it said it was when it actually came to putting the money on the table. In an interview with the Trust chief executive in 1995, she confessed that the initial difficulties were in providing information to the purchasers. However, they also felt that they were treated rather condescendingly by the purchaser, and were not accorded the same status as other Trusts. In addition, she recognized a division within the purchasing authority between those in public health who had a clear idea of what CHS were and supported them, and those in finance and contracting who appeared not to reflect that message.

The provider did not think that there was anything particular to CHS that made them difficult to specify in contract form. As the provider director of contracting put it:

> 'I think there are a lot of things that can be measured in community, and I think we should start with those and get good data on that . . . You can measure. You can measure a reduction in hospital beds to correspond with increased activity in community. You can measure the uptake of vaccinations. You can measure the number of children detected before a certain age with difficulties. There is a whole range of things you can measure.'

As far as she was concerned it was the provider who should lead on this because they had the 'expertise on the services', although this might alter as 'people learn in purchasing'. She saw CHS as providing specialist expertise in the community, interacting with primary and social care, and that it was important that this expertise was recognized, and not just seen as what happens when you get out of hospital.

For the purchaser, however, focusing too much on the paperwork of specifications and contracts obscured the way in which the fundamental issues were cultural rather than contractual. As one purchaser manager argued: '. . . changing the way in which services are delivered is as much about changing professional practice and professional mind-sets as it is about any sort of contract or anything which is written down on paper'. While the purchaser should have a clear direction about where services need to go, and be good at specifying what the service should entail, they had tended to approach it informally with providers, in an 'interactive process'. The definition of services, on this view, is not something that can be done in abstract and defined and contested in a contract, but has to be part of an evolving collaborative relationship. Whatever tensions and conflicts may emerge at senior level, it was important to keep the work going at the clinical interface even though in terms of contract prices, that would involve only 'minor influences on a major contract'.

Area 2

In Area 2 there was much uncertainty about the likely shape of both provider and purchaser organizations, and the prospect of considerable organizational turbulence. Individual DMUs were bidding for Trust status, but there was also talk of a larger 'city-wide' Trust. The area consisted of three separate health authorities and a family health services authority, but it was increasingly clear that some kind of merger was imminent. In spite of attention being diverted by these issues, purchasers and providers both felt that CHS posed problems for the 'managed market', although the reasoning underlying this perception sometimes differed.

In a working group report on the organization of community health services in the area, eight 'key principles' were identified as of major importance to the organization of CHS: strategic planning and policy formulation; interagency coordination; professional standards; responsiveness to local needs; capacity for evaluating response to need; avoidance of duplication of services; and recognition of client preference for a 'seamless service'; and recognition of the focal role of the GP. On this basis, the working group concluded that '. . . a city-wide organization should be set up as soon as it is practicable, characterized by a central body and local provider executives'. It also noted that while some of these principles might be achieved by 'centralisation, others will depend on which is close to the people for whose services it is responsible'.

There were, however, many difficulties involved in the development of a city-wide Trust. The three community units in the area were all organized very differently. While they all had 'basic core services' common to each of them, the level and range of services varied: the unit of management under which the services were organized differed (in one district the service was managed from hospital as outreach while in another it was provided by the CHS and liaison arrangements were set up with the hospital); each district CHS had numerous schemes and projects which had grown from responses to particular local circumstances. While all three districts had district nursing and health visiting, only one had special school nurses and elderly care teams, while one other had elderly screening and a stroke rehabilitation team.

The organization of CHS for the provider did not easily lend itself to corporate self-presentation. This was illustrated by the director of community health services in an integrated hospital and CHS Trust:

'There are actually a number of strands, a significant set of which fall under primary care . . . which covers district nursing and health visiting . . . It also includes community orthoptics, community dietetics, community medical services . . . [and] . . . all of the services relating to immunisation . . . That group, the total set, is something like 250 people with a budget of £4.3 million. Separate from that there are a number of other services that have a community focus. There's psychology, which is separate from psychiatry. There's speech therapy and chiropody, and learning disabilities.'

While purchasers were often preoccupied with other more pressing financial issues, on the provider side the likely shape of CHS and their place in contracts was more salient. The contracts manager from Area 2, working for what became the first CHS Trust in the region, described the view from the centre in 1992 as being that CHS were not able to stand alone, and he argued that region were unable to grasp the complexity and the potential of independent CHS units. This is not surprising when one considers that the DMUs themselves were trying to come to grips with what sort of contracts were likely to be usable in relation to CHS: quality of services, packages of care, cost-and-volume contracts and so on. The contracts manager expressed the degree of uncertainty surrounding CHS at that time:

> 'Really we're trying to *re-define* what we are. We may provide some highly specialised services (for example, learning disabilities), some managed agencies (for example, therapists) sold back to hospitals and GPs, and then some core work, bread-and-butter services (like district nursing), sold to the health authority purchaser.'

Within one of the other constituent health authorities, where there was an integrated acute and community Trust, CHS were seen to be 'at a *very* rudimentary stage', according to the Trust director of planning. Information on CHS was lacking, and the content of the services varied for each of the city's three health authorities. For example, the district in which this Trust was located had community midwives and community psychiatric nurses managed by the community Unit General Manager, but this was not the same elsewhere. In general, the relationship between hospital services and CHS was still unclear and subject to change. Moreover, the director of planning could foresee problems over the specification of CHS because of the 'variety of forms of provision and split responsibilities . . . It is very difficult to measure the output and outcomes of CHS when deciding what to purchase and provide. This is because of multi-agency involvement, all providing different quantums of care.'

By the autumn of 1992, the purchasing plan had been approved by the DHAs, and more detailed documents had been produced which would provide the basis for negotiation and agreement about the exact services required of providers. It is at this point that we begin to see evidence of more intense analysis of the nature of services and the problems involved in contract specification. The purchasing consortium in Area 2 which had been formed as a halfway house between three health authorities and a fully unified commission, was beginning to grapple with how to begin to move resources from the hospital sector into the community health services, and, therefore, how to develop new CHS specifications. According to the consortium's director of contracting, they wanted to get providers to think about what services were needed, what direction to go in, and what resources are required.

Interesting differences of opinion regarding the extent to which CHS pose particular problems for the workings of the internal market then emerged. For the consortium director of contracting in Area 2, the nature of contracts and the process of contracting transcended any substantive differences that might be said to exist between different kinds of services or different sectors of service delivery. He could see no difference, for example, between contracts with the voluntary and the statutory sectors. As far as he was concerned:

> 'We are interested in health problems and health care, not CHS *per se*. The organizational boundaries between primary/community/secondary are *irrelevant* from the point of view of us as purchasers.'

Moreover, in view of the standardization brought about by the contracting process, he did not think that there was any difference in principle between CHS and acute hospital services. Community services are not distinctive because they have multiple clients, needs and professionals, he argued (look at general medicine or surgery) and there is no qualitative difference between acute and community health services. For this reason:

> 'It is not intrinsically difficult to specify CHS. It is the lack of information, data, that is the key problem. It is an informational issue, *not* a conceptual issue about the nature of the service.'

The draft purchasing plan had focused on hospitals and they had not made much advance in specifying CHS:

> *Interviewer:* How do you 'track' CHS elements in contracts?
> *Director of Contracting:* Through DHA papers – the service specification should be there.
> *Interviewer:* But most of those we've seen are effectively one-line statements.
> *Director of Contracting:* Yes. Often that is all there is for CHS. It's a reflection of the lack of information. District nurses or health visitors simply tell you the number of visits made; we don't know the purpose, the client, or the outcome.

The consortium chief executive echoed these sentiments. However, he did think that while the problems of specification applied to both acute and community health services, there were other ways in which CHS posed particular problems. Community contacts were less easily identifiable than FCEs, 'the ECU of contracting' as one Trust director of contracting dubbed it. And furthermore: 'The concept of CHS is very different from other types of health – it's about an ethos or culture.'

Part of the culture of CHS is related to the locations and the way in which it is delivered. Competition between services is more difficult to envisage. Whereas with acute hospital services there will be a variety of accessible suppliers, and the main criterion for choosing to do business with one rather than another is price:

> '[W]ith community services and care, dealing with the housebound in most cases, the *only* way is for competition to come from selecting providers to come to the patient's home. In practice this is not very easy, to imagine competing providers.'

Thus, for the purchasers in Area 2 there are a number of ways in which CHS pose difficulties for the contracting process. These can be summarized as problems of conceptualization, information and location.

For the providers, the picture was a little different. The specification of CHS was more than a matter of defining a service. It was, as we have seen, a more profound question of identity and purpose. The nature of the process of defining services was of importance to many of those working in specialties which could fall on either side of the fence dividing hospital and community. Psychiatrists, for example, but also many professions allied to medicine, were fighting against being moved into a free-standing CHS Trust because they felt that their professional strength would be 'diluted', and that their prestige and status depended upon their being part of a hospital. The question of defining 'community' and 'hospital' is, therefore, not at all as clear-cut as one might expect. In the period leading up to the development of what became the city-wide Trust, there were many 'turf-wars' fought over which services could be located where and with what implications. Those with a more managerial agenda were keen to define as 'community' anything which took place beyond the island site of the hospital Trust.

Many of the problems over meaning and definition emerged from discussions about 'information'. In an interview with the contracts manager for the community trust, it was evident that there were '. . . problems over information generally'. Some of these problems were technical, to do 'with producing more meaningful measures of performance', as the Trust contracts manager put it. 'We're still developing our activity data, based on quarterly contacts. For example, district nursing, there are terrible problems in producing this.' And later he added: 'This problem of volume and workload is not yet settled. The difficulty is measuring district nurses, health visitors and other activity through patient contacts.'

Other aspects of the information problem were more political. For example, the purchasers wanted information on overheads and skill mix – information, that is, about the resources with which the providers were working and exactly how they were using them. The provider felt that the purchaser should only have information on activity levels. In February 1993, in a meeting between the consortium and the community Trust, it became clear that the Trust was not happy to provide the level of information the consortium was requesting:

> 'We're not prepared to accept this, especially information on grades and levels of staff. You're looking for information on activity and outcomes surely.'
>
> (Trust chief executive)

> 'We as purchasers need staffing data to check activity data, because it's meaningless. To judge trends, we need data . . . We also need to check contact hours to monitor contracts.'
>
> (Purchaser director of public health)

> 'I firmly believe this is *not* an appropriate measure; the only measure we have is activity. There's a serious issue here about how much monitoring is being required.'
>
> (Trust chief executive)

Eventually, as the two sides struggled to hammer out the contract for 1993–4, they settled to agree on activity at 1992–3 levels. It was clear that the matter of what sort of information should be made available to the purchaser by the provider was left unresolved.

At this point, the city-wide purchasing consortium was still contracting with the three districts yet to be unified into a city-wide Trust. However, only one of these districts had a clearly defined separate community services Trust. The other two had some kind of integrated service in which community service issues were not discussed separately.

In Area 2 at this time, the consensus of opinion within the purchasing organization was that community services did pose particular difficulties for the commissioning and contracting process. However, it was less clear whether these difficulties were to do with the amount of information, the quality of information, or the nature of the services themselves and their location. The director of contracting in a combined hospital and community services Trust said that the process of contracting had '. . . been driven by the needs of elective surgery. Contracting is all number counting with money attached to throughput'. Nonetheless, it was felt at this time that some kind of measure of CHS activity was necessary.

Organizational uncertainties had ontological consequences for the roles and identities of the people involved. Mergers were probable for both purchasers and providers, but it was not at all clear who would be merging with whom, and a number of different plans were in existence. In the words of the community Trust contracts manager: 'We're sailing into the unknown . . . People are increasingly aware that we are going into a no-man's-land . . . The merger issue is dominating senior managers'. At the same time, the purchasing consortium were grappling with how to move towards full-scale merger. An additional big issue from the purchaser's point of view was how to improve the health of the population with less money available.

For both purchaser and provider, CHS were an important consideration in the developing relationships in the local internal market. For the purchasers these services were not, in principle, more difficult for the contract mechanism than any other kind of services. It was not a conceptual but an informational problem. For the providers, in contrast, there was the feeling that their services were different, and were posing difficulties for purchasers at this time. These services were culturally distinct, and for this reason they posed difficulties of conceptualization and definition which were not open to an easy technical solution. As the chief executive of an integrated hospital and community Trust argued: 'CHS are not really in a competitive environment. The nature of the services are such that they've got to be local.'

Area 3

Fieldwork began in Area 3 in the spring of 1993 shortly after the contracts for 1993–4 had been signed. The health authority and the family health services authority were joined as a single organizational unit with a view to becoming a commission along the lines of the national 'standard bearer', Dorset Health

Commission. As far as the chief executive was concerned, they were 'rewriting the script'. On the provider side, the community unit had become a 'shadow' Trust with effect from April 1993. This comprised maternity, mental handicap, learning disabilities, children's services, community nursing, and paramedical support (with physiotherapy being split with the acute Trust).

Area 3 differed from the other two areas in having a more blurred division between the activities of the acute and community Trusts. From the outset there was much more open competition for services, and, at least as far as the community Trust was concerned, wariness at any sign of favouritism to the acute sector by the purchaser. While the community Trust retained some acute services, such as some services for the elderly, the acute Trust sought to diversify its provision in, for example, physiotherapy, outside the hospital walls. As we will show, this problem over the definition of community and acute services led the purchaser into particularly close relationships with the community Trust in negotiations over efficiency savings and contract prices. In financial terms, the contract with what became the community Trust was slightly larger than that with the acute Trust.

Like Area 1, Area 3 had a very strong strategic framework for contracting to achieve 'health gain' for the population of the area. Early on in the fieldwork, the chief executive indicated that his main interest was in the 'integration' of services, and he manifestly had little time for the tidy separation of 'acute' and 'community' services. While recognizing that CHS did potentially pose problems of information and measurement, he did not want to get mired in what he clearly saw as distracting details. For him the key strategic question was: 'How can we use money to do things better? We have to break away from the institutional model. It's about boundary shifting.' This desire to shift things around and be more integrative, combined with the fact that the locality contained a much higher proportion of GP fundholders, meant that Area 3 differed in having a much closer relationship between the developing 'commission' and GPs (both fundholders and non-fundholders) than was the case in the other two areas.

In 1993, as the community division was becoming a Trust, the community directorate was larger than any in the surrounding conurbation. The clinical director informed us that it included community nursing (health visiting, district nursing and various specialist nursing groups), clinical psychology, occupational therapy, dietetics, the community dental service and the adult learning disabilities service. It had over 800 staff and had work going on in 23 health centres and clinics, as well as all the hospital sites in the locality. With such professional and geographical diversity, a corporate image and plan was difficult to develop, and there had always been 'potential conflict' between the central management and the service heads over decisions regarding investment and disinvestment. The clinical director argued that each area of the CHS needed to develop its own niche marketing – palliative care, for example, was a niche involving a variety of different services. This high-profile marketing, a contrast with Areas 1 and 2, was partly related to the much higher level of the purchaser budget held by GP fundholders.

The problem of information about CHS was important in Area 3 also. In 1993, the clinical director for CHS told us that there was 'nothing in the community' (by way of information technology), 'everything is paper and pencil . . . information is a massive problem for us, massive'. While the provider recognized that their community-based work was poorly specified in terms of activity and contact data, it was also felt, by the provider director of finance, that the purchaser was really quite happy to roll over the contract from the year before with something for inflation, without reference to details. They were interested more in 'quality' than activity, whereas some other purchasers were more interested in the details of activity. The lack of sophistication lay in the purchaser's expectations more than the provider's techniques. With the main purchaser representing approximately 70 per cent of the provider's income, there did not seem to be much pressure to increase the sophistication of the internal monitoring procedures.

Many, but not all, CHS were seen to pose problems for the contracting process because of difficulties in specifying activity. According to the provider clinical director:

> 'It is for health visiting, not for district nursing . . . you can almost itemize the activities of district nursing . . . They've got activity codes to record their activity against objectives . . . Health visiting is very much more difficult to specify in terms of activities.'

It was also seen to be difficult because of the multi-agency working that necessarily took place around managing complex health problems in the community. And this was especially so in the context of a stated philosophy of 'empowerment', again according to the provider clinical director:

> 'There are areas of community services which are not easy to delineate, where different agencies have to work together. That's in the nature of community services: community health, social services, the voluntary sector, primary care, the acute sector, all interface with each other; and there has to be a degree of consensus . . . and a complex model of service delivery. Especially as the professional model that we use is one of empowerment. Empowering individual families and communities to develop and take responsibility for their own lives. It's not the same as having your leg put in plaster.'

From the provider's point of view, this agenda was largely shared by the purchaser, but when it came to contracting there were difficulties in mapping specific services onto programmes of care, and programmes of care onto health gain. During 1993–4, as the purchaser began to look at what it wanted for health gain, this lack of fit between purchaser and provider became more a source of tension, as Chapter 6 shows.

It also became increasingly clear over the fieldwork period that 'community services' as used in purchaser documents such as the purchasing plan, were not necessarily synonymous with the CHS directorate in the Trust. Further growth in community services, from the purchaser's point of view, might mean looking for efficiency savings (cost-improvement programmes) *within* the provider's existing budget rather than the purchaser coming up with new money for growth. While the provider recognized the financial problems they might face, and the reality of competition over the therapy market from community outreach from the acute Trust, for the community nursing services there was, according to the provider director of finance, a limit based on more than the weaknesses of the information base:

> 'I think in most of the areas it's going to be difficult to see any real competition. If you think about our elderly service . . . children's services, most mothers don't want to take their children long distances, they want to go somewhere locally . . . Community services [too], again you're going to want somebody that is local and can provide a fast service.'

It was also recognized by the provider, however, that the high level of GP fundholding in the locality might create pressures as fundholders began to look more closely at the skill mix and 'try to obtain better value for money' (provider contracts manager) and to some extent this informant considered that the Trust was increasingly being 'driven by the GPs' agenda'. Fundholders needed information, and the Trust was becoming increasingly aware that reliable information about levels of community services was inadequate, 'a black hole' (provider contracts manager). This was particularly true of community nursing, and less so with more highly specified areas of activity such as chiropody and dietetics.

During 1993, the purchaser in Area 3 considered in more detail what CHS were about, and what qualities they should be seeking to support. The purchaser director of finance recognized that 'localness' (purchaser director of finance and contracting) was an important quality of CHS. While this did not mean that they would always contract with the main provider, it did mean that the only factor that would lead them to contract with another provider was where they are geographically closer to residents living at the edges of the health authority's territory.

In seeking to move from a community contract which was 'just one line with one sum of money' (purchaser director of contracting), the purchaser was attempting to break away from a definition of services that was set by the provider. In pursuit of health gain, what the purchaser wanted was to develop a 'seamless' service. It did not matter whether residents were getting care from health-care workers based at the acute Trust, or the community Trust. The purchaser strategy, therefore, was to contract for community health services, not to contract with this or that provider. Nonetheless, the conflict over 'ownership' of services provided in the community was a problem. The following exchange between two purchaser contracts managers, one responsible for community and one responsible for hospitals, illustrates this:

> *First purchaser contracts manager:* There is a danger of setting up more and more specialties in nursing, and there is the problem of the interface between specialist nurses and community nurses. This raises the issue of ownership with the consultants wanting to keep hold. There is a real danger of creating specialists in the community.
> *Second purchaser contracts manager:* The consultants want the hospital outreach work in urology. We need to evaluate it. I'd want to be treated by a specialist nurse.

First purchaser contracts manager: But we don't want to create specialists
who are not needed. There is often no justification for specialists, and
we don't want outreach to be a hospital service.

In order to break down the gap between the global concept of 'health gain' on
the one hand and on the other the reality of numerous services provided from
different sites, the purchaser attempted to develop two purchasing strategies.
First, a strategy based on care group analysis: '. . . if we start off from the focus
of our residents, what we want is to purchase something that has all that group
needs' (purchaser director of finance and contracting). The second strategy
was one of locality purchasing, or at least 'locality-sensitive purchasing' (purchaser community contracts manager), based on a detailed understanding of
the overall health needs of particular localities in the population using information from GPs and local user and voluntary organizations. While there
might appear to be potential conflict between these two strategies, a crucial
role was played by the health strategy managers in Area 3 in helping to dis-
aggregate the 'community contract' into care groups and reconfigure it in
terms of locality health needs, working with the 'contracting team' to develop
contracts appropriate to locality needs.

The purchaser also recognized, however, that none of this could be done
without adequate information systems. Towards the end of 1993, the quality
of information about CHS was, in the words of the purchaser director of
finance and contracting, 'non-existent: What we need really is the development of the information systems that give us community contacts . . . We
need to develop those information systems, and first of all we need to develop
the data collection to see if it actually tells us anything about the service.'
Although the purchaser declared itself committed to the shifting of resources
from institution to community, it was predicted that the problem of information would show itself more strongly in the next year when block contracting
would come to an end, and the purchaser had to demonstrate what it had
spent its money on. Also, increased activity in the community was taking
place, regardless of the origin of the services being delivered in the community. The health-strategy managers were seen to play a crucial role in generating more adequate information about what was taking place on the ground,
and to feed this back into the contracting process.

In Area 3, therefore, the definition of CHS differed between purchaser
and provider. The former had a very clear population focus on health gain,
and any particular provider units – acute or community – were seen as
serving the production of health gain. What they required from the provider was flexibility, and information about services against which to look
at the effectiveness of their strategy. For the provider, there was some
tension over the relationship between the services they provided and those
of the acute hospital trust. While they were keen to be responsive to both
the main purchaser and fundholders, they still defined their activity very
much in terms of specific, dedicated services, staffed by professionals with
particular skills. This difference provided the basis for the conflicts which
we discuss below.

Conclusions: community health services in a turbulent environment

While the problem of defining the form and content of CHS has always existed, with a tendency to define them residually, the process of contracting requires far greater clarity. However, at the very time that one aspect of the reforms was leading to an insistence on the need for clarity, other aspects of the organizational environment were making specification of CHS much more difficult. Alongside an understanding of the importance of CHS came the realities of power play within health-care environments which meant that the new CHS Trusts were competing for resources with their much more powerful counterparts in hospitals who had greater political visibility. The problem of conceptualizing CHS was more than a technical aspect of contracting. It raised fundamental questions about the philosophy and values of care, and about appropriate organizational forms for services so deeply embedded with the networks of local relationships.

This uncertainty was most clearly exemplified in Area 2, but was also evident in Areas 1 and 3. The director of contracting for Area 2 told us that during a particularly fraught period in 1994, negotiations over services were 'slipping away into something else':

'We have reached an understanding of the *services* we're contracting for, [and have] drawn up various lists and schedules . . . but the main issue is over *resources*.'

The details of the resource issue are dealt with in Chapter 6, but it is important to recognize the impact of this upon the definitional issues relating to CHS. In view of the financial pressures upon the amalgamating Trust, and the possibility of their having to cut or 'rationalize' services, the purchaser came to have a more urgent interest in discussions of exactly what the services were and their relationship to resources.

The turbulence in the financial environment raised important issues for the provider Trusts about the organization and measurement of what they were doing, and the extent to which different community services could be defended in a politically sensitive environment. Apart from the differences between districts in what counts as a 'contact', and the difficulties this posed for identifying 'real' as opposed to 'artefactual' differences, there were also variations between services, with health visiting being much more ambiguous in information terms than district nursing. For the Trust in Area 2 there was the feeling that '. . . the ME [Management Executive] outpost and the region don't understand the complexity of community activity . . . They are under pressure to tick boxes and get value-for-money . . . [and compared to acute services] Community is a growing irritant and becoming a problem' (Trust director of contracting and planning).

It was a problem which drew in many interests. The purchaser continued to insist that there was no difference in principle between acute and community services and that the same kind of 'incentives and penalties' should be applied. The region wanted proof of efficiency, while the Trust director of contracting and planning maintained that '. . . it is difficult to measure CHS in those terms,' and that efficiencies in the acute sector had an impact on CHS: 'We say that CHS are not like hospital FCEs: hospitals can increase their productivity by earlier discharge, but that simply *decreases* our productivity.'

The response of the purchaser and provider managers in Area 2 was to set up a 'strategic liaison group' to respond to crises over resources. Throughout 1994 and into 1995 this group entered into detailed discussions over finances and how '. . . to unpick the overall community contract, . . . breaking it down into smaller contracts, giving them some more definition, and moving towards agreement at the level of services. We want to unpick the generic community services . . . It's much better to have joint discussion on services and priorities' (purchaser chief executive). Starting with 'easier ones' such as 'family planning' and 'learning disabilities' it was recognized that '. . . work should also start on the more complex ones including community nursing' (purchaser director of public health). At the moment: 'We have no idea about the current disposition of nursing services across the city, its volume and range. It's a closed book' (purchaser director of contracting).

By the end of 1994, there were still problems for the Trust officers in knowing what 'efficiency' could mean in CHS in the absence of any agreed contract 'currency'. Also, the Trust continued to insist that CHS posed a major *conceptual* problem for the workings of the market, while the purchasers, although recognizing that definitions do not just reflect 'real' work, still felt that 'some measures *are* valid, so we shouldn't overgeneralize' (purchaser director of community care). During early 1995, therefore, the purchaser was still looking for improvements in information from the Trust so that it could assist in prioritizing services, while the Trust felt that the purchaser did not understand the peculiarities of CHS. Underlying all the detailed discussion about costs and activity, therefore, there was a profound analysis unfolding of the nature of the community health services and their place within the NHS. There was, in the words of the purchaser director of contracting, a 'gap in understanding between us and a gap in substance'.

The relationship between the political economy of resources and the semiotics of CHS were most sharply evident in Area 2; but they featured too in the other fieldwork areas. In Area 3, for example, the battle over the meaning of community services and information about community services became increasingly strenuous as the purchaser attempted to contract efficiently and effectively within regional resource reductions. During numerous meetings between the protagonists, discussions about resources and cash became the vehicle through which differences in definitions of community, measures of activity and the nature of information were strongly debated. While the purchaser wanted to base their efficiency targets on community contacts, the provider complained that it was difficult to use this information as the basis for comparing different services because there is no standard currency for CHS, and '. . . we cannot add up apples and pears' (provider director of finance). Even within particular specialties, such as community nursing, the situation was one of chronic uncertainty over how to enter a dialogue over something which could not easily be disaggregated, defined and measured. At one meeting, the purchaser director of finance and contracting exclaimed: 'I'm coming to the humble realization that you don't know what you're selling us, and we don't know what we are buying. We're all just pretending.'

During 1994, the negotiations between purchaser and provider were 'very much a battle about money' (purchaser community contracts manager). But behind this battle were more profound philosophical doubt and political uncertainty about the nature of CHS and how to match services to population needs. After the 1994–5 contract was finally signed, the provider director of corporate development still confessed: 'We never did clearly define what was meant by community health services.'

In this chapter we have shown how the definition and measurement of, and information about, CHS have underpinned debates over contracting between purchaser and provider. CHS do pose difficulties for the operation of the internal market, but there are variations in the amount of difficulty posed by different CHS. In Chapter 3 we look in more detail at the culture of commissioning and contracting, and examine some of the ways in which the conceptual and cultural differences posed by CHS work themselves out in the commissioning and contracting process.

3

Health needs and

outcomes in the

contracting process

The history of the response to the NHS reforms by social scientists and health-care workers is one of movement from wholesale criticism to uneasy accept-ance of parts of the package. This may reflect a change of heart – being co-opted into a certain kind of ideological framework – but it may also indicate the extent to which the many reforms and their multiple effects simply cannot be rolled back to reveal a pristine 1948 or even 1974 version of the NHS. Eight years on from *Working for Patients*, it is now a package with many parts, and there are differing degrees of scepticism with regard to their likely effects on the health of the nation. While, in general, many continue to regard rationing or cost containment as the heart of the programme which has unfolded since 1989, it is also recognized that there were many undesirable features to the system that existed at the start of the 1980s, such as bureaucratic rigidity and professional dominance, which some aspects of the wave of reforms since the 1980s have helped to break down.

One aspect of the reforms which has engendered considerable consensus across the political spectrum is the emphasis on the assessment of health needs as the basis for purchasers' decisions about health and social care. In the wake of the Acheson report on public health in England (Acheson 1988), the re-sponse of the Department of Health (1988) signalled the direction in which the health service would have to go:

> It is widely recognised that the provision of health services should be informed by an assessment of health needs in the Region or District

concerned, combined with evaluation of the extent to which services provided successfully tackle those needs.

The attempt to link needs to services and services to outcomes, through the contracting process and by other means, is something which is generally regarded as an advance on the system as it was – driven more by the ambitions of the medical profession than the needs of the populations served by the NHS (Pickin and St Leger 1993). Health needs assessment (HNA) and the evaluation of outcomes are important platforms of strategic planning in the NHS, and a means of challenging those paradigms and interests which have traditionally dominated the health services (Small 1989).

The desire to evaluate the effectiveness of health services by linking needs and outcomes is also market-driven in so far as it represents an attempt to track and control the use of resources. However, it is also seen as a way of making a professionally dominated service ultimately more responsive to those who need and use it by making purchasing decisions, and thus the services provided, more tied to sound evidence about needs (Popay and Williams 1993; Popay and Williams 1994b). Assessing needs and evaluating outcomes are tasks which are necessarily contested, and especially so in a quasi-market.

In the context of the shift towards a primary care-driven, community-oriented NHS, the stage is set for a real struggle between the commissioning authorities, the growing numbers of fundholding GPs, and the traditional bastions of medical power in the teaching hospitals. This is not a simple matter of breaking down monopolies through opening up the market. After all, many of the changes taking place in the acute hospital sector, particularly in London, have looked more like traditional public sector planning than the operation of markets. Nonetheless, the emphasis on services based on need and evaluated in terms of their contribution to health gain at the population level, clearly poses a threat to the traditional power balance within the NHS.

In our three areas there were varying degrees of attention paid to HNA, on the one hand, and the monitoring of outcomes on the other. In Areas 1 and 3 (see Appendix) there was a clear philosophy of population health gain, although there were differences in the way they attempted to link this into the contracting process. In Area 2, much health needs work seemed to go on, but with little apparent linkage to the contracting process. In all three areas, however, there was a sense of difficulty in relating the broad strategic aspects of purchasing to the specifications involved in the contracting process. For some this meant that health needs and health gain were little more than rhetorical terms employed to justify contracting intentions. For others, on the contrary, strategic decisions linked to health needs and health gain were more real than the contracting process which, as we will show later, often involved little more than one-line contract statements about district nurses or health visitors. In this chapter we discuss the processes of linking needs to contracts; contracts to outcomes and to population health gain. In Chapter 4 we look in detail at the extent to which local people were incorporated into this process.

Health needs assessment and contracting

The areas

Area 1

The purchaser in Area 1 had a strong political commitment to, and a clear philosophical framework for, HNA. In 1992, the chief executive explained to us that the health authorities saw the purchasing process as linking needs to resources and resources to outcomes. Within this process, access to some resources was achieved through contracts, while for others it was done by other means. There are many informal sources that contribute to meeting health needs which would not be part of formal contracting for health services. For this authority, whatever difficulties there may be over details, the important thing was to keep in view the goal of health gain for populations. This was a view with which the CHS provider concurred at that time, seeing themselves as working 'closely with the purchaser' whom they saw as the regional 'leader'. An emphasis on outcomes, therefore, as we indicate below, was central to the discussions in this area.

In a purchaser paper, the goal of HNA was defined as: 'To support decision-making by recommending options based on information about health problems, health resources and health outcomes in order to target resource distribution and improve health.' It also specified three elements to the processes directed at this goal: the provision of sufficient relevant information, the appraisal of options, and supporting decision-makers in targeting resource distribution.

However, HNA was not seen to be the purchaser's sole prerogative. The provider in this area was keen to have its expertise in local knowledge about health needs recognized, and to be involved in the HNA process, but at the start of 1993 this was not happening, and the provider indicated that although they had expertise in HNA, they could understand that the purchaser might see it as 'the tail wagging the dog' if providers were too closely involved in HNA. However, in relation to decisions over prioritization and investment in specific services, such as audiology, the purchaser well understood that although '. . . we are supposed to be the needs assessors, [. . .] we need expert advice, so it's not that simple'.

The aim in Area 1 was to operate as a team in which HNA, led by public health consultants, fed into the work of the contract team: 'We don't build up barriers between ourselves [. . .] We see ourselves as purchasers first, then concentrating on certain areas second' (purchaser contracts manager). A public health consultant bluntly informed us: 'I can't just stick with community services', because within the population model of HNA, the services themselves were secondary. Talking about services set up a 'false boundary'. For many of those working in Area 1, even talking in terms of client groups was seen as a diversion from the focus on the population, assessment of whose health needs was supposed to drive the service.

The public health consultant recognized that HNA should feed into contracting but that there was bound to be a delay. HNA in any one year would not feed into the contract for that year, or even the year after:

'The process is for me to do the needs assessment, then feed into contracting. Really, you need a two-year gap to do the needs assessment,
then following on with the contract, which is why it has been difficult
over the last two years (1991–3) – we haven't had the needs assessment
to feed in.'

The process they wanted to put in place was one where social and health-
services purchasers would be able to use the health needs information to say
what services were required, match these to resources, and define the outcomes that they wanted to achieve. The 'health needs' people in the health
authority would then sit down with the contracting group about the practicalities of how this might be achieved. As far as this informant was concerned
the problem was not in relating health needs to contracts but 'service development'. They were finding it difficult to shift the providers – not surprisingly
perhaps – from a service-driven ethos to one more responsive to health needs,
and this was put down to the fact that they were 'medically dominated' and in
a 'monopoly position' in relation to the provision of particular services,
though this was much less the case for the community services than for the
acute sector.

The purchasers in this area recognized the tensions between different developments in health policy which cut across the simple logic of population
HNA feeding into contracting for health gain. As the public health consultant
responsible for health gain told us: 'I'd prefer not even to look at client groups,
I'd rather just look at population groups, but we're forced into it because of
Health of the Nation, things like that.' This meant there was a tendency to
define health needs 'in terms of what is available'. The contracting officer for
the authority pointed out that in seeking to develop partnerships with providers at the grass roots, they inevitably worked with particular services organized around specific professions with their own roles and identities – 'they
reflect how community in services are organized'.

At this point in 1993, therefore, population HNA orientated towards health
gain was a guiding philosophy, but one which its proponents were having to
compromise in order to respond to all the other developments taking place in
the health service. 'This organization can't wait for me to do all the needs
assessments' the same consultant said, towards the end of 1993, 'they can't
hold still for twenty years. The Government is already insisting on all kinds of
things that we have to do.' But without the developmental, needs assessment
work, he warned, we would see a return to 'the old decibel planning stuff'.

During 1994, the discussions between purchasers and providers became increasingly difficult as they tried to reconcile the health-gain philosophy with
purchasing specific services organized in a certain way in the context of
nationally and regionally imposed financial limits. During a meeting in the
summer of 1994, the following exchange occurred:

Purchaser chief executive: We need to improve information about demand, and improve our needs assessment. If we freed up £100K next
year . . . what is your priority service?

Provider chief executive: It would be OT (occupational therapy), and then speech therapy for adults with mental health problems
[. . .]
Purchaser chief executive: But what about the *effectiveness* of OT? How can we show that?

In spite of the difficulties involved in reconciling the differences between the needs-led and services-led approaches to contracting, the strategic view within the purchaser remained clear. 'We don't *focus* on CHS', as one health strategy manager put it, '[. . .] the new agenda is to use HNA to influence cost-effective planning based on *need*'. Moreover, during 1994 there were small areas of success for the authority in developing needs-led purchasing. In the area of eye care, for example, they managed – in the teeth of much resistance – to shift money away from cataract surgery into the rehabilitation of people with macular degeneration. A needs-led approach was also developed in relation to 'sexual health', where it informed a decision to disinvest from existing family planning services in order to encourage a reconfiguration of those services. These real shifts in resources caused profound anxieties in the provider even though the investment decisions were, according to the purchaser director of contracting, a 're-direction' as opposed to a 'pulling out' of resources.

For both purchaser and provider in Area 1, 1995 was a year of considerable change. The health authority and the FHSA were merging with their equivalents in a neighbouring authority and were to become a commission from April 1995. This necessitated major internal reorganizations of the management structure, and consequent role and career uncertainty among many of our key informants. At the same time, both purchasers and providers were continually being hit by a regionally imposed priorities and the development of primary-care-led purchasing.

It was in this turbulent situation that a new strategic management team was set up in January 1995. During the first of these meetings, attended by senior purchaser managers, reflecting on the enormous turbulence now evident, the purchaser chief executive had to remind the meeting: 'Needs assessment is a health authority priority: the long-term work goes on at the same time as the day-to-day work.' However, there was still scepticism in the Trust about the extent to which the circle could be squared. This can be illustrated by two interviews with senior managers, one from the community Trust the other from what was by this time the health commission:

'I think the people working on health needs assessment and service development in purchasing have no insight at all into contractual arrangements, and don't link their proposals to any sort of contractual agreements; they merely talk about developing A, B, C, D and E without any reference to contracts, income or money. They talk about outcomes, but they don't talk about contracts.'

(Provider chief executive)

'I think that in the areas where we have done some quite in-depth needs assessments [and] strategy development work this has had a significant impact on the way that services are delivered. [. . .] In some ways we've jumped from producing a strategy to talking to the clinicians. It's only at a later stage that we've actually drawn up a service specification. [. . .] I'm coming round to the opinion that changing the ways in which services are delivered is as much about changing professional practices and mind-sets as it is about any sort of contract.'

(Purchaser health strategy manager)

The two informants agree that contracting is at the centre of the purchasing process. However, while the provider sees the purchaser's unwillingness to move from strategy to contractual detail as an impediment, the purchaser sees the contract as to some degree marginal to the strategic objective of changing services and achieving health gain.

Significantly in Area 1, the provider saw a division within the commission between the finance and contracting officers who understood their requirements, and the health needs and service development officers who seemed to be unable or unwilling to engage with the particulars of the contracting process. We will see a similar situation in Area 3. However, in Area 2, the situation was far more tense in political terms, and the publicly amicable relations which were preserved in Area 1 were less in evidence.

Area 2

At the start of our project, the district that we call Area 2 was represented by three DHAs serving populations with very distinctive histories, cultures and socio-demographic characteristics. After merger, it comprised deprived inner-city localities and affluent suburbs. For purposes of HNA, the locality represented a challenge to purchaser commitment and ingenuity even in times of resource gain. However, this was a time of significant resource loss due to the application of per capita funding reductions.

On the provider side, there was the development of a city-wide CHS provider with some outreach and other work operating from other centres. In abstract terms, the relationship between the different components of the purchasing process was seen to be simple enough, moving through a familiar and well-rehearsed cycle: health needs assessment → preparation of service requirements → specification of contracts → contract monitoring → evaluation of outcomes → health needs assessment. However, the details of the process depended very much on local circumstances. For the purchasers in Area 2, the merger process provided a context for thinking about health needs. It was recognized that the increasing size of the purchasing authority necessitated a different approach to HNA. From the viewpoint of a district general manager in 1992, it was to have four zones, each doing 'local voices' type work and linking up with the FHSA and the CHS workers.

For providers too, the implicit model employed was one of 'joint health needs assessment':

'CHS pick up the local knowledge quickly and identify them earlier than purchasers. District nurses and health visitors are good qualitative

researchers, and inform locality managers of local needs and problems –
they really know what's going on in their patch. Purchasers don't have
this degree of detailed knowledge, or pick up on local changes and their
context.'

(Provider contracts manager)

For community services in particular, information about needs 'resides in local
staff' who are in a position to develop 'locality profiles' (provider general
manager). However, the providers also recognized that information was most
valuable in the context of a quasi-market, and sharing it went against the
'essentially competitive situation'. Moreover, the provider had to be aware of
the purchaser's requirements for information for the purposes of contract
monitoring in addition to HNA. For this reason, the desire to share information and collaborate in HNA had to be tempered by a sense of *Realpolitik*: '. . .
the key thing is health needs assessment – we can help the purchaser, but the
issue is how much information we should provide. The information is one of
our marketing tools' (provider contracts manager).

By the middle of 1993, as far as the business and contracts manager of the
CHS provider was concerned, 'the relationship with the main purchasers is
[. . .] one of partnership. Things are laid back, and we are into a developmental
phase'. However, as many of the providers recognized, for all the talk of partnership, 'at the end of the day the purchasers have got a strategic view of the
direction of health care in the city' (provider director of community services).
By the start of 1993, purchasers were confronting the problem of how to link
the general statements of policy objectives laid out in the purchasing plan at
the end of 1992 with the 'specific services required from providers' (purchaser
director of contracting). This informant's broad conclusion at the time was:
'You can't!,' and the purchasing plan statements were really a platform for the
'process of negotiation' required to make the connections with specific units
or services.

'We are interested in health problems and health care not CHS *per se*. The
organizational boundaries between primary/community/hospital are
irrelevant from the point of view of us as purchasers.'

(Purchaser director of contracting)

However, in view of the fact that CHS can be seen to represent what one non-
executive health authority member called the 'professionalization of the
everyday', it was not expected that the purchasers would talk tough with the
CHS providers. Rather, they would use their 'familiarity' with the services to
open up a process of negotiation for changes in service delivery.

As the three health authorities became drawn together in a consortium,
therefore, the key issue was how to relate the development of a purchasing
ethos based on health needs assessment to the specifics of the contracting
process. The chief executive of the purchasing consortium recognized that the
approach adopted in Area 2 was 'more mechanistic' than in some other areas.
He argued that if you ask purchasers what they wanted from CHS '. . . it was
rare to get any explicit or crystal clear spelling out of needs' (purchaser chief

executive). He recognized that the problem of linking needs to outcomes was found across all services and specialties, but that there were less identifiable measures of output in CHS, 'no hard-nosed, definite outcomes'. This made CHS contracts more uncertain than those for acute services.

In this area, therefore, both the purchaser and the provider expressed an interest in the process of HNA and linking this to contracts. The CHC, too, recognized that HNA assessment was an area of work in which it could build up relationships with purchasers alongside its more traditional relationships with the provider. The CHC recognized that they did not have the resources to get involved in any full-scale needs assessment themselves, but they could make an input to the work being done by the purchasers. As the chief officer of the CHC put it: 'We're flagging up areas of unmet need and saying this is something that should be looked at, but we're not in a position to do that in any depth ourselves.'

Discussion of HNA and its relationship to the purchasing plan during 1993 indicated uncertainty about what the process should encompass – where it should begin and where it should end – and difficulty in relating broad discussion of public health issues and concerns about how to 'prioritize' to specific items to be contracted for and purchased. For example, in discussing the relationship between HNA work and the purchasing plan in May 1993, the following exchange occurred between three members of the Purchasing Strategy Forum:

> *Assistant director of contracting*: We should have detailed descriptions of each service first.
> *Consultant in public health medicine*: No, that is a service specification.
> *Director of contracting*: We're looking for the end result, recommendations for the plan.
> *Consultant in public health medicine*: [We must have] issue, [then] recommended action [then] resources.

In a similar way, in relation to the action plan for *Health of the Nation* targets, the consortium chief executive asked with a touch of exasperation: 'Are there two or three things we can say we are actually *doing* for each objective? Within the purchasing plan can we put actions that we can actually do, and link them to contracts?' The answer given was that you could only do this if you referred to resources which would then require further justification as to why certain spending priorities had been decided. Beyond the difficulties of conceptualizing the process whereby information collected through HNA would feed into the purchasing plan and then into contracts, discussion at the meetings also contained a reflexive understanding of the ethical and political framework of the process in which they were embedded.

The issue of resources was seen as being in profound tension with the whole concept of a needs-based service. At one meeting, for example, a public health consultant argued firmly:

> 'Priorities come from a *needs-base*, rather than from reduced resources. We as an organization have accepted that we are *more needs-focused*. Then we'll deal with the dilemma of resources.'

Health needs assessment was seen to play a critical role in preventing 'arbitrary decisions' being made on resources and services. As the director of contracting put it, again with considerable force:

'If we don't have linkages between services and resources and the health needs work, we'll have missed an opportunity. *We're here to get that linkage.*'

At this meeting there was no direct disagreement with this view, but there was a recognition of the difficulty in seeing HNA as a simple bulwark against resources-driven arbitrary decisions on priorities. In response to the director of contracting, the chair of the forum added:

'Health needs must be in focus, but we must also address problems and service changes which have a health needs dimension. It's a complex problem of prioritizing the overall list [. . .]. There are implications which are not health needs *per se* . . . the horrendous problem of resolving externally-imposed demands and internally-generated demands.'

Moreover, it was also recognized that in the process of HNA, things may emerge from the people's expression of preferences on priorities which did not fit with the strategic views of the purchasers. As one public health consultant asked rhetorically in the wake of a recent 'local voices' initiative on the priorities for children's services: '*Which* things will we protect? Community services and priority services? These may not come out from the consultations.'

Encased within these purchasing strategy forums, and emerging in situations such as the one we have described, was an uncertainty and an anxiety about the nature and extent of purchaser power within the reforming NHS. There was a constant wariness about slipping back into what was referred to on more than one occasion as 'old NHS-speak', meaning that the purchasers were not flexing their muscles enough with regard to decisions on priorities and were allowing things to be driven either by national regional decisions or by the *status quo ante* of power within provider organizations.

It was within these discussions about health needs and service prioritization that the complexities of the 'managed market' emerged most clearly, as the needs-driven perspectives of purchasers who had examined 'market demand' came into conflict with national, regional and professional sensitivities over the shifting of resources away from hospitals into community services. At another meeting discussing an agenda item on the implications of per capita funding, the director of contracting pointed out that community services costs were 'above the regional average', but another officer replied: 'I don't think the figures are meaningful. They don't relate to needs.' However, the chief executive then reminded the meeting that 'need has to be squared off against finite assumptions'.

A profound difficulty emerged for the purchasers in this area, of how to honour their commitment to shifting resources from hospitals to primary and community services in a way that was linked to an assessment of health needs, without causing a decrease in hospital activity. As far as the CHS providers were concerned, they saw the reduced revenue allocation as a betrayal, and felt that the purchasers saw them as a soft touch because of their low visibility and the difficulty in demonstrating that they were meeting health needs.

During 1993 in Area 2, it became clear that in spite of the needs-led policy of shifting resources to primary and community services, the purchasers were having difficulty in sustaining that in the face of pressure from providers, from region (concerned with the political implications of withdrawal of funding from hospitals), and, indeed, from members of the authority who (for whatever reasons) remained committed to hospital care. Some officers were increasingly arguing for equal treatment for hospitals and community services, while others, such as the purchaser head of nursing services insisted that 'the hospitals' arguments about "health" must be challenged. We will invest in *general health*, not treating illness and elective surgery'.

It can be seen, then, that arguments from the principle of health needs formed an important component in more detailed discussions over finance and activity, and that purchasers would need evidence that health promotion and CHS were the best ways of improving the health of the population, against the interested scepticism of the hospitals and acute specialties. From the purchaser's viewpoint, it was increasingly important that the community trust had 'an information strategy in which we can believe, one that is genuinely shared and owned by both of us' (purchaser director of contracting).

In this regard, the purchasers in Area 2 compared themselves unfavourably with adjacent authorities where it seemed that there was a much more explicit and clear strategy for health improvement based on a consistent argument about the need to shift resources away from the powerful hospitals. The director of contracting for the still autonomous FHSA argued that the consortium had not yet developed a 'perspective on the best configuration of services' and was therefore 'still reactive to events'. The purchasing plan, she argued, had to be more than the process of contracting, entailing an overall strategy for the development of services in the locality. But it was difficult not to be reactive in the context of the financial pressures. The 'bottom line', as far as the Director of contracting was concerned was that, in the context of the per capita funding, '£9.3 million *must* come out, mostly from hospitals – and *that's* the issue'.

During 1994, the difficulties of tying HNA to contracts continued to be recognized as a problem for purchasers. As a purchaser public health consultant indicated:

> 'HNA has many definitions – it's not just about health measurement, but also option appraisal. It's not just a question of collecting data and proceeding from there. Health needs assessment is difficult, especially for community health services. CHS has never had the attention focused on it that acute has – the data available is much worse, very vague.'

The purchaser, it was claimed, was aiming to be more needs-led and needs-based, but the contracts were still conceived of in terms of services. This made it difficult to incorporate the kind of user-led health needs assessment that many of the public health team in the purchaser wanted. How could they show that local voices initiatives were taking on board what people said if the services were remaining the same?

The recognition of this strategic difficulty in reconciling, among other things, a health needs-driven system with one orientated to professionally driven, specific services with increasing regional pressures to achieve indicated 'deliverables' underpinned the development in the summer of 1994 of a special joint group in Area 2 bringing together the chief officers of the health authority and the Trust. This group was increasingly driven by the need to monitor and manage the impact of service reductions and, consequently, with the necessity to understand what the outcome of these reductions would be on 'deliverables', as discussed below. In the context of this 'strategic group', the task of forging imaginative strategies for health gain came to be an ever more distant project. They were so preoccupied with the pressures brought about by reductions in the regional allocation, that more long-term thinking was difficult. At the same time, however, the director of contracting for the purchaser argued that that pressures did mean that for CHS '. . . now there is beginning a serious discussion of priorities. We're asking: "what are we going to have to de-prioritise?"'.' In these situations, those, such as the director of nursing, who tried to remind the meetings that '. . . we need to be aware of our health needs assessment and the population morbidity' were often drowned out in the cacophony of concern over immediate political and financial issues, as Chapter 6 shows.

There was a profound problem of what senior managers referred to as the 'currency' of CHS. What did they mean by 'efficiency', 'activity', 'outcome', 'meeting needs'? And all these uncertainties were being discussed within the pressures from region. In this context the relationship between needs and activity in CHS was a complex one. As the provider chief executive put it: '. . . If the greater work we do is due to increased patient *dependency*, our activity (in the sense of numbers of contacts) will drop: in meeting needs you'll get less activity.' The purchaser chief executive retorted: 'We know that the efficiency index distorts work and distorts priorities, but it is your job as managers to reconcile meeting needs with central government expectations.' For both re-sources and activity, these issues revolved around crude arguments about frac-tional changes in percentages of growth in money or volume of work.

Alongside the harsh discussions in these so-called 'strategic group meetings', there were parallel discussions operating with different discourses. There was a purchaser group discussing strategy which produced and discussed papers on fundamental issues to do with how to improve health services in the area. While this meeting involved some of the same personnel, the atmosphere and the orientation was quite different. In one paper produced for a meeting at the beginning of 1995, a section on 'the health needs of local people' argued: 'We need to start with something on the health and needs of local people, that we then drive through to implications for services: partly to deflect the argument that the whole thing is resource driven; partly to establish the credentials of the health authority as being here to serve the population.'

Many of the discussions at these meetings were about how to convince 'the public' that beds and bed reductions and ward closures were not the issue and that the health services for the area had to be looked at more broadly and more imaginatively. 'How do we make this convincing to people?,' argued a public health consultant somewhat rhetorically, to which someone else responded: 'I can't even convince my family!' It was recognized that this was not surprising in view of the widely held perception that the commission had 'caved in' to pressure from the large, powerful hospital trust in the area. It was also recognized that grand plans for the health services of the area inevitably implied commitment from other organizations over which the health authority had no jurisdiction and little influence. They were supposed to 'commission' on behalf of the area and to organize themselves to do that, but in situations of alliance with uncertain partners.

Area 3

Area 3 contained a highly innovative purchaser working as a unified commission long before it was formally recognized as such. Moreover, the purchasers were also keen to work with GPs as purchasers and providers, and, through the system of health strategy managers, with the front-line CHS provider staff. There was perhaps a clearer sense than there was in Area 1 of how to link an overriding philosophy and strategy of health gain with the reconfiguration of services into 'programmes of care'. However, there was still some anxiety in the provider Trust, in 1993, about some of the 'avant-garde community projects' (provider clinical director, community services) to which health visitor resources had been re-allocated from general practice.

From the purchaser's point of view the 'avant garde' was simply a reflection of the 'locality sensitive' approach to purchasing that they had a policy to pursue. Being locality sensitive meant: '. . . try to listen to GPs, local groups, and forge links with the community, influence our purchasing decisions by the information coming up through grass roots – listening really' (purchaser contracts manager, community services). While the philosophy of health gain was very similar to that in Area 1, Area 3 purchasers seemed to have a more fully developed sense of how to develop that through locality working. In some ways they were less sure of how HNA assessment would develop:

> 'I think we're very good at bringing in all the players in looking at the service and seeking views, but what we've not developed is the more hard-nosed health needs assessment aspects of epidemiology, outcomes research.'
> (Purchaser contracts manager, community services)

The Trust, however, saw itself as having a key role in the HNA work in the area. Indeed, at the end of 1993, the provider director of finance thought that the purchaser relied 'to a very great extent on its providers to inform it about where needs are'. This had partly emerged as a consequence of the very good working relationship that had developed between the purchaser, and the director of public health in particular, and the providers of CHS on the ground. It was also significant that many of the personnel on the purchaser side working as 'locality managers' had backgrounds as CHS providers.

As in other areas, however, it was felt that the purchaser was less rational in using the purchasing plan to inform contracting than it sometimes claimed. As far as the Trust director of finance was concerned, they did not get '. . . the kind of considered well thought-out analysis of needs assessment and review of existing resources that would result in a specification and a budget allocated to a particular service'. He thought that the key managers in purchasing were excellent at 'thinking', but 'hopeless at implementing it'. This sense that the purchaser was not following through the purchasing plan became sharpened in the debates over finance that took place early in 1994, and a growing distrust of both parties, one for the other, as Chapter 6 shows.

The Trust felt that the purchaser was not switching resources from acute to community at the level they had been led to expect. Part of the reason for this, one senior manager at the Trust suggested in a contract negotiation meeting, was that '. . . it's harder to commission community health services'. From the provider's point of view, a lot of the work that had gone into matching needs to resources and then built into the purchasing plan was never really put into effect. This had created difficulties for the provider whose business plan was driven to a large extent by their expectations of the purchasing plan. As far as the purchaser director of public health was concerned, however, this was shifting the responsibility. As far as she was concerned, it was the responsibility of the purchaser to decide on the strategic vision for the change of services, but '. . . it's the responsibility of the provider to deliver on that vision'.

One of the features of purchaser activity in this area was the way in which the emphasis on and activity with *localities* meant that there was a continuing relationship between purchasers and providers at levels other than those between senior managers at the point of contract negotiation. Through locality managers, accountable to the director of public health, the commission had set up neighbourhood health strategies which involved the locality managers working closely with the provider community nursing services in public health advocacy. This neighbourhood strategy work, along with the work of public health nurses in HNA, created lines of relationship between purchaser and provider which lay outside the contractual relationship. According to the purchaser chief executive, the ultimate aim of this kind of extracontractual relationship was to link up with primary care, and have the GPs and the public health nurses routinely conducting HNA in which they would be supported by the commission, and to whom they would pass information on.

The commission had also been concerned to develop an approach to HNA and purchasing that opened up a role for users, which we explore in Chapter 4. This was the time when the then health minister, Brian Mawhinney, was 'majoring on user involvement', as the chief executive put it. However, a recent evaluation exercise involving a team of management consultants had been disappointing in this regard, and in an interview in 1994, the chief executive felt that in organizational terms it was '. . . not working to a tightly ordered structure that links the involvement of users to the production of our plans, and gives them a direct opportunity to influence the plan'. He felt that the reasons for this failure were partly to do with the fragmented and heterogeneous nature of the 'users', and that historically the system is so driven by organized professional interests.

The future of health needs assessment

The general conclusion of our investigation was that HNA had not yet been related in any systematic way to contracting. The perception of there being no structured relationship between HNA, the purchasing plan, service specifications and contracts was a dominant theme in our interviews with key officers as they reviewed the experience of the two contracting rounds we had observed:

> 'The purchasing plan objectives somehow got sort of lost when we got to the negotiating table. [. . .] I think it was a very frustrating experience, having tried to do some work on health needs . . . it was an academic exercise really, because it *didn't* link with the process of contracting, and the contract discussions didn't link to the promotion of health.'
> (Purchaser director of primary and community care)

The future for HNA, this key informant argued, lies with the purchaser developing and extending its role as a networker, and not relying on the community Trust 'as the only voice of the people':

> 'I think the wealth of expertise and knowledge is already here in this locality, but not necessarily embodied in community health providers as we currently see them. There are lots and lots of people out there who look after themselves in all kinds of effective ways, and we need to tap into that. We've got high unemployment here, we've got responsibilities to our own citizens to create some job opportunities as well.'
> (Purchaser director of primary and community care)

It was clear from the interviews we conducted that the problem of HNA was closely tied to the attempt to develop more meaningful evaluations of the health outcomes or health gain achieved through the commissioning of services. It is to the problem of outcomes and the development of outcome-related contracts that we now turn.

Towards outcome-related contracts

Area 1

Commissioning for health gain was a mantric phrase for the purchasers in Area 1, and was central too to the provider's perception of the roles and objectives. The provider business and contracts manager in early 1993 wanted to 'make the contracting process more outcome-oriented':

> 'We have to learn to make this big jump from thinking about services to thinking about outcomes, but it is a slow process, and will probably take longer than we first thought.'

Part of the reason for this, it was suggested, was that it is difficult to assess outcomes clearly: 'CHS,' she said, 'are "inadequately measurable".' Moreover, while outcomes might be theoretically definable, the reality was that the process of purchasing for health gain did involve working with client groups and localities as well as with outcome objectives specified in terms of population health gain. Nonetheless, the importance of this overall perspective was reiterated time and again, by purchasers in particular.

Service agreements for CHS were seen by the purchaser as 'a meaningless exercise' and what was needed was an outcome and quality orientation to the contracting process. However, this was difficult to achieve in the absence of input from comprehensive population HNA which, as we noted above, could take a long time to feed into the contracting process. Information from the purchaser was a serious problem: 'We have no way of knowing what is going on in the community,' a public health consultant said. With health visiting, for example, the purchaser had no idea what the provider counted as a contact. 'They may be talking to the parents of the child under five about a whole range of things, about family planning, about safety, about lifestyle, all kinds of things, we have no idea.' However, there was a danger of focusing too much on the quality of information about *services*, when the major problem, from the point of view of Area 1 purchasers, was HNA.

Although the provider in this area declared itself sensitive to the health needs and health gain agenda, they also felt driven by other pressures. The chief executive was concerned about what areas of service to cut in a situation of reduced funding, recognizing that they '. . . have to invest in those services we're going to attract income from. We have to look at key services we want to promote.' These conflicts of view were still apparent in the spring of 1994 when the business manager of the community Trust told us: '. . . purchasers are interested in telling us what outcomes and what sort of services they want, not how those services should be delivered.'

As we indicated earlier, the purchaser and provider moved slowly and incrementally to the development of services based on HNA with meaningful 'measures' (loosely defined) of outcome. Near the end of our fieldwork, informants looked back on what had been accomplished and noted a sense of development. As the director of contracting for the purchaser said of the contract with the community unit for the treatment of leg ulcers:

> 'If they get the community provision wrong more people will go into hospital. [. . .] If they get it right fewer people will go into hospital. We've got an outcome measure, and we can stipulate healing rates both in terms of percentage of patients and time. Now that's the kind of contract we need to develop. A quarter of a million district nurse contacts tells me sod all.'

Although the purchaser was perceived by the provider as being an organization with two arms which did not necessarily agree, or know what the other was doing, this comment from the director of contracting suggests that there was a common agreement on the importance of defining outcomes as the basis for developing better contracts. The emphasis on the contract was not one that the purchaser and the provider in Area 1 shared, although whatever they thought in private in public the meetings were negotiative and reasonable. In Area 2 the situation was different.

Area 2

At the other end of the commissioning cycle was the problem of how to monitor and evaluate the quality of the services delivered, with both purchasers and providers recognizing that there was a long way to go on the pathway to genuinely outcome-related contracting. Nonetheless, the beginnings of this process could be seen in the increasing pressure felt by the providers from purchasers who were '. . . getting more sophisticated in requesting *quality* indicators' which the provider had in the form of patients' satisfaction surveys, clinical audit and various outcome measures. The next step for the providers was to improve outcome and patient-dependency measures, with the main focus being work with district nurses, locality managers and service heads. For example, in community-based physiotherapy, they had developed 'six outcome measures' using professionals' judgements. For the provider this was very much work that the purchaser *required* them to do.

During the course of 1993, the main CHS provider was having to produce monthly returns to the Department of Health on finance and activity, the latter being described for the most part '. . . in one line in numbers of patient contacts'. They were also having to provide the main purchaser with information quarterly, the ME was monitoring their business plan, and the zonal outposts wanted quarterly verbal reports and 'good news, bad news' summaries. Not surprisingly, this provider – like many others no doubt – was feeling overstretched. Also, this information actually did not mean very much in terms of quality of outcomes. The provider was very aware of their limitations at that time. 'It's down to our professional services,' a contracts manager told us, 'to identify what are meaningful dependency measures and outcomes for their area of work'. But he confessed that their data systems were inadequate at that time.

The director of quality for the consortium recognized the difficulty in producing outcome data for CHS, but she felt that the fragmented nature of the services allowed them to set up small-scale, imaginative models of good practice which could be looked at in terms of health gains and outcomes to provide a firmer foundation for future specification of contracts. While contracts and specifications had not yet been based on such analysis of services against needs,

> 'I think we will see in the next couple of years the development of fairly easily transferable measures around outcomes for service. I don't think they are easy to identify because the interventions are more complex. The benefits and effects are not as obvious, and are longer term. [. . .] We're looking at measuring the health of a community over a longer period of time, and we're certainly looking at different responses in different communities, so we should look at different measures.'

As far as the director of quality was concerned, intellectual energy had to be put into this, and the process should not focus on conventional measures of need and performance. Traditionally, community interventions had been 'overprofessionalized' and that non-professional, 'community development'-style interventions needed to be explored.

From the purchaser's point of view, the provider seemed, at the end of 1993, to be failing in its obligation to make available adequate monitoring information. The provider chief executive pleaded that they '. . . hadn't got the capacity'. This was not enough for the purchaser:

Purchasing director of contracting: Is there disagreement that quality objectives should be focusing on quality in community health services?'
Provider contracts manager: There is a difference of opinion on what we're
using as the major currency of quality.

There were pressures also from the region to see 'results' quickly, with attention
being given to 'crude productivity indices' – total number of contacts divided by
the total number of staff – which the provider contract manager thought to be 'a
ridiculous measure'. Nonetheless, looking to the future, they were developing a
'minimum contract data set' based on nationally defined 'care objectives in
order to make the contracting process more realistic in the sense of being more
outcome-oriented'. Throughout 1994 there were expressions of tension between
the provider claiming to want to think creatively about CHS and the pressures
from region through the purchaser to have 'performance', and a growing insistence on 'quantitative and measurable indicators' to measure 'deliverables'
which were politically and publicly popular. The provider Trust felt that this led
to 'softer' aspects of performance being ignored which worked 'against CHS as
they are configured': 'In community services it's difficult to show that you are
getting more for the same, or less, resources' (provider contracts manager).

Ensuing discussions revolved around more and more detailed methodological
excursions into the basis on which it could be said that the provider was doing
more, or less, or the same for what amount of money. It became apparent that
the purchaser wanted not just measures of performance in simple activity terms,
but some understanding of the quality of what was being provided, with the
provider pointing to the existence of a 'quality group' who would be dealing
with information problems in that area. There was also a growing appreciation
of the heterogeneity of CHS, and the need to 'unpick the community contract'.
While the aim was to have some 'measurable output of outcome for each service'
(purchaser chief executive), it was also understood that this might be easier for
family planning or physiotherapy than it was for health promotion.

Looking back in the summer of 1995, however, the purchaser director of primary and community care argued that the measurement of effectiveness or outcomes was no more difficult for community than for acute services. Most measurement in both hospitals and community was crude activity or contact counting –
response times, waiting lists, case mix. True measures of outcome or quality,
indicators of clinical effectiveness and appropriateness, were not being monitored.
However, she suggested that this was now what they were trying to do:

'We are doing some work on outcome measurements, and you can do
this even for community – things like infection rates, pressure sores,
length of treatment times for varicose ulcers. All sorts of things that tell
you whether it's a modern district nursing service or a traditional one.
But there is a long way to go.'

Area 3

As with our two other fieldwork areas, both purchasers and providers were
concerned with how to demonstrate the quality of what was being provided as

an outcome in CHS, particularly for community nursing. The Trust head of community nursing acknowledged the size of the task: '. . . we can try to do work on dependency coding and some outcome measures, but generally it is beyond us. But we have got to get to grips with this.' Meanwhile, the health authority director of finance and contracting told us, as had many other purchaser representatives in our other areas, that counting 'contacts' for district nursing or health visiting '. . . doesn't tell us anything; our needs are beyond that'.

The development of meaningful information for contracting was a priority for purchasers. The purchasing plan for 1993–4 indicated their intention to collaborate with the provider in developing outcome-oriented contracts. They were starting to develop what they saw as appropriate outcome indicators in specific, defined areas. In one of the purchaser's operational contracts group meetings towards the end of 1993, the contracts manager with responsibility for CHS told her colleagues:

'We are all working to outcome-oriented contracts. This is a development issue [. . .]. I want a good honest discussion with providers . . . There is already a family planning contract in existence, but we've not signed it. There are 'outcome' measures, but they are largely 'process' based. There is little on actual knowledge of outcome in terms of pregnancy . . . There are lots of issues around outcome measures – should we use subjective measures, such as patient satisfaction, or objective measures, such as rate of wound healing?'

One of the purchaser health-strategy managers, however, was sceptical about the readiness of the authority to work with outome-oriented contracts, while supporting the philosophy. She felt that they were 'a bit ahead of themselves,' and that outcome-oriented contracts 'were not going to be a reality for a while yet . . . we need some stepping stones to that'.

The providers were quite positive about outcome-oriented contracts. Indeed, according to the business manager for the community Trust, they led the way and then 'shelved it due to the complexity of it. [. . .] It was becoming increasingly complicated, and we weren't too sure just what enthusiasm the purchaser had for it'. The provider now wanted to develop programmes of care, with outcome measures attached, though the business manager also recognized that it would be a long process especially when 'the word "outcome" means different things to different people'. Nonetheless, in terms of the development of more sophisticated models of contracting, those services with more clearly defined outcomes would be at the leading edge.

There was a danger, however, recognized by both purchaser and provider, that developing more sophisticated contracts through outcome measurement might become an end in itself. Indeed the provider director of finance told us that 'outcome-based contracts have become rather a cliche'. He went on:

'. . . the rationale being that purchasers should not be involved in looking at numbers of health visitors, whole-time equivalents. What it should be doing is matching its resources to need, and what matters is whether needs are met, not how they are met.'

At a theoretical level, both purchasers and providers would find nothing to disagree with here, but from the provider's point of view, there was a danger that the purchaser would get drawn more and more into matters of operational detail, in spite of their commitment to the broad needs, resources and outcomes model. As far as the provider was concerned, the development of outcome measures was important, but it had to be seen as *development* work.

Nonetheless, for the purchaser, the ideal monitoring tool for CHS was the outcome-oriented contract, but the outcome '. . . has to be one which doesn't lie within the power of the health service to mimic' (purchaser director of public health). On this basis, death is a 'good outcome' as is teenage pregnancy, and for CHS it was important to construct some kind of 'hard measures'. These could be statements of patients' rights which the purchaser would contract to meet, or a set of hard outcomes – a case of measles is a poor outcome of a measles vaccination programme. However, in the hurly-burly of contract negotiation and monitoring it was recognized that '. . . it's difficult to demonstrate health gain – it's such a wide subjective concept' (purchaser director of finance and contracting).

This continuing uncertainty among at least some of the commission's directorate, along with the inevitable difficulty for the provider in reconciling their provision of specific services with global concepts of health gain, led the chief executive to feel, in the summer of 1995, that they had not really succeeded in 'getting to sort of common ground on what the new NHS agenda really is'. He felt the commission were fully behind the whole move towards evidence-based decision-making in the NHS. They want to know '. . . what contribution this or that change will make in health-gain terms. It's outcomes we're looking at. The response we got from the Trust missed that point completely'.

From the outside, however, there did not seem to be as much distance between commission and Trust as this excerpt would suggest. In two 'exit' interviews, the commission chief executive told us: 'My view . . . is that we really need to try to concentrate our effort on identifying some outcome measures.' The chief executive of the Trust suggested: 'There's very little work being done on outcome measures. We started some work a while ago on programmes of care that's never gone anywhere [. . .] and that's how we would like to sell our services.' It seemed to us that the differences were discursive. It might be too strong to say that the Trust and the commission were speaking different languages, but there were certainly developments to be undertaken in exploring the frameworks within which they were operating in thinking about needs and outcomes.

Conclusion

In this chapter we have looked at the relationship between HNA and the contracting process, and more briefly, we have examined the concern among both purchaser and provider organizations in our three areas about how to develop more adequate and meaningful assessments of outcome. We have suggested that the systematic use of analysis derived from HNA in purchasing plans, service specifications and contracts, has been limited in all three areas. In part, these limitations are caused by difficulties in connecting global issues to do with health needs to contracts for specific services. They are also due to the turbulence in the NHS which has introduced regional and national initiatives into the system, making it difficult to match resources to needs in any systematic way.

We found that both purchasers and providers placed considerable importance on developing the technology and skills to facilitate more effective HNA and outcomes evaluation. There seemed to be some uncertainty about who was best placed to do this work, with purchasers claiming the larger strategic overview, and providers claiming more detailed information about health needs derived from regular patient contacts. Although providers inevitably saw things to some extent in terms of existing service configurations, this did not mean that the Trusts in any of our three areas were blind to the need to make services responsive to needs.

It seemed to us that the process of linking needs, resources, services and outcomes was one that required much closer linkage between purchasers and providers. The most successful examples were in Area 3 where the purchasers had stepped outside the contractual relationship between senior managers in order to cultivate collaborative network relationships between intermediate-level managers in the purchaser organization and service heads in the provider Trust. It was here that the face-to-face work of service development for improving the health of the population was taking place, and it was here too that the flexibility required to develop meaningful outcome measures was most clearly understood.

4

Local voices and

community health

services

The dominant objectives of the NHS reforms have been fiscal and political: to control public expenditure on health care and to challenge the power and autonomy of the professions working within the health-care system. However, an important ideological argument providing ethical justification for these objectives has been that the NHS needs to be more responsive to the needs and preferences of potential and actual users or consumers of health services. A central thread running through the rhetoric of reform has been that greater managerial control over professional work and enhanced provider competition in the provision of services will give consumers more choice and more control.

With the introduction of the internal market, the expectation was that health authorities would take more account of the views of local people in their commissioning and contracting strategies. Alongside the traditional emphasis on the consumer voice at the point of provision, therefore, there was increasing consideration of how local people, as users and potential users of services, could have more input into all phases of the commissioning cycle.

Many commentators have drawn attention to the difficulties involved in realizing this vision of a service responsive both to consumers and resident populations. As Deakin (1993b: 1–2) points out:

> To be fully effective these internal cultural transformations need to be matched by a fundamental reorientation of the perception of the users of public services; they must be persuaded to regard themselves as customers and behave as such.

This is not necessarily going to be a simple transformation, not least because of the difficulties in applying consumerist assumptions of active, confident, un-stigmatized behaviour to the realities of health service use (Barnes *et al.* 1990: 109). The application of consumer principles to public services may be inherently problematic. As Potter points out (1988: 150): 'The resources of the public sector are finite and limited, and distributed as an act of political will. This creates an immediate dilemma for the pure application of consumer principles.' In contrast to the situation in the private sector, equity considerations mean that the interests of individual citizens must be balanced against the interests of the community as a whole and the interests of one group should not be enabled to take precedence over the interests of another group, so that there could never be unfettered individual 'choice' even if resources permitted it. Potter further points out that while consumerism may be a helpful concept in encouraging authorities to think of individual members of the public, not as passive clients, it does not automatically turn members of the public into partners involved in the planning and monitoring of these public services.

In view of these doubts about the applicability of market concepts to health-care services, the term 'users' is often preferred to consumers (Barnes *et al.* 1990). Consumerism does not necessarily contain within it the condition that users have a high degree of control over the services they receive. Moreover, 'control' may be exercised at a number of different levels, right through from informing through partnership, to delegated power and citizen control (Arnstein 1969).

Different purposes may lie behind the differing levels of involvement of users, with two categories of intent being discernible: (1) those which seek to improve the quality of services by making them more sensitive or responsive to the needs and preferences of individuals who use them; and (2) those which seek to extend the capacity of users to participate in decisions about the design and strategy of services (Barnes and Wistow 1992). Underlying these categories of intent, of course, is the imbalance of power that exists between professional providers of services and those who use them. As Plamping and Delamothe (1991: 204) comment: 'Clearly stated individual rights might benefit the powerful and articulate, but they will not do much for those who lack the means to negotiate for their own health.'

Local voices

Whatever the ideological limitations of the concept of a user-responsive health-care system, the consumer has been a key motif of the reforms since the publication of *Working for Patients* (Department of Health 1989a) and the importance of 'listening to local voices' has been a specific emphasis within the Government's statements since 1992 (DoH 1989d; Hunter 1994; Popay and Williams 1994b; Donaldson 1995).

In January 1992, the concept of local voices was etched clearly on the map of health-service reform when the NHS Management Executive published a document entitled *Local Voices* in which it was argued (1992: 3):

To give people an effective voice in the shaping of health services locally will call for a radically different approach from that employed in the past. In particular, there needs to be a move away from one-off consultation towards ongoing involvement of local people in purchasing activities.

In this document, 'local people' was used loosely to refer to a representative cross-section of individuals, groups, leaders of opinion and voluntary organizations. Involvement meant a combination of information-giving, dialogue, consultation and participation in decision-making, and feedback. A speech by the then Minister of Health in April 1994 declared that (NHS Executive 1994: 12):

'We must get away from the notion that health services can be designed for the community by "experts" who define people's needs but ignore their "wishes".

The Minister called on health authorities to involve the locality in both a preliminary consultation about what should go into a purchasing plan and a formal consultation on a draft plan.

On the provider side, while NHS trusts do not have a statutory obligation to consult on proposed changes to services, the National Consumer Council (1992) points out that good relations within the local community make for a more effective service and in all provider units, the quality of service can best be judged by the users and their carers themselves. The *Patient's Charter* was directly geared to provider units, but the 'local voices' idea was a purchaser responsibility. However, the boundaries are increasingly blurred. Many consumers are unaware of the distinction between purchasers and providers (Popay and Williams 1994b), and some provider units, particularly for community health services, may regard themselves as being more in touch with the needs of local people than are purchasers.

User involvement and its limitations

User and carer groups, and voluntary organizations in general, are important channels through which local voices can make themselves heard. Voluntary organizations can be distinguished in various ways: some of them are provider organizations, some are deeply engaged in campaigning or advocacy, some are user-based, some relative-carer based, and some are a combination of all of these. As a result of the changing culture in the NHS, several voluntary/user groups are evolving from pressure groups into providers of services. For some, the event of becoming the main or sole provider organization in their field could mean, for example, that they are able to deliver a culturally appropriate service for their particular client group, and the new role of main or sole provider can thus empower the voluntary group in its relationship with the statutory authorities.

There is, however, an acknowledged possible source of friction between the need to maintain independence and the need to generate income, and while advocacy appears to be a crucial part of what everyone is doing, nevertheless, according to a representative of a local branch of a large national voluntary group, 'the whole issue of monitoring and advocating on behalf of the [users] then brings you into potential conflict with the same authorities with whom you are negotiating the contract'.

During 1993–5, formal contractual relationships between health authorities and voluntary groups in our fieldwork areas (see Appendix) were rare, and the involvement of, and consultation with, local people and users has to be looked for at other points in the commissioning process. In order to understand the perceptions and experiences of user and patient representatives, this chapter presents qualitative evidence from the case-study areas.

Users and community health services

One of the major difficulties of CHS, both from the perspectives of managers and service users, is understanding what they mean. CHS are difficult to define and, therefore, troublesome to enumerate. They taper off into hospital-based services at one end and social services at the other. This ambiguity has its roots in history (Lightfoot *et al.* n.d.: 33):

> For community health services, a satisfactory operating definition of health has long been a problem. The problem is derived largely from difficulties of clarifying the respective boundaries of health and social care.

This continues to be reflected in the difficulty many service users have in comprehending that some of the CHS they may receive are controlled by the health authority and not social services. Most of our respondents – purchasers, providers and users – seem to fall back on the tautology that community health services are those services provided by CHS units. These services will vary in particulars from one provider unit to another – some may include community mental health services or midwifery, for example, while others will not. But there will also be a core of services common to most units – services such as district nursing, health visiting, orthoptics, audiology, speech and language therapy, chiropody, physiotherapy, dietetics and clinical psychology. The difficulty that arises, therefore, is that although the purchasing and provision of CHS is of vital importance to local people, it is very difficult for local people to have clear information about services available.

In the following, we therefore examine evidence for the extent to which local people are brought into the commissioning and contracting process.

Local policies for local voices

Health authority policy documents produced in the fieldwork areas demonstrated a firm commitment to 'local voices'. For example, in 1992, the purchaser in Area 1 commissioned a survey in which '[T]he intention was not simply to list people's opinions of specific health services but to explore the values and beliefs underlying those opinions'. The purchasing board followed up this survey with an attempt to formulate a policy on using local voices in purchasing. In this area, therefore, the clear intention was that local people should be involved in planning, health needs, and prioritization or rationing. The needs of local service users were also to be taken into consideration upon the advent of any policy or structural changes within or across localities centred in the region.

The purchasing plan in Area 2 for 1994–5 stated that one of their aims and objectives is to 'listen and respond to local people and to empower individuals and communities so that they can take action to improve their own health'. On the provider side too, there was evidence of considerable commitment to the idea of local people's involvement. Trust business plans within Area 1 and Area 2 all contained statements of commitment towards the principle of involving local voices or adhering to the *Patient's Charter* as a means of taking into consideration the views of service users.

The commissioning or purchasing cycle is divided into a number of stages and there is no reason why public participation could not occur to some degree in all of these stages. Purchaser documents indicated that the intention was to involve 'local voices', but what evidence is there of local people influencing decision-making at different stages in the commissioning cycle? We will consider this from the points of view of purchasers, providers and users.

First, however, we must understand the purpose which purchasers perceive to lie behind involvement of users in planning health-care services. Several views emerged from interviews with purchaser managers across all three field-work areas. These included: the need to comply with statutory requirements; the perception that people have a right to information and to know how their money is being spent in a tax-funded public service; the desire of health commissions to obtain ownership of decisions by being seen to make them with the support of the public; and the wish to arrive at better decisions and thereby obtain better services.

There were, however, acknowledged limits to the idea of user involvement from the point of view of managers. The first was that there are finite resources and a necessity to inform users that, while their opinions are wanted and valued, there were financial constraints. The user or lay perspective is only one of a number of perspectives to be taken into account when health-care decisions are being made. At the same time, there were confusions and ambiguities surrounding the purpose of user involvement. Purchaser managers in all three areas confessed that they were often not clear about whether they were consulting with a view to the public having a major role in determining the outcome, or consulting with the view to simply making their decision better informed. This confusion regarding the ultimate purpose of user involvement has also been found in other health authorities (Goss *et al.* 1993; Lupton and Taylor 1995).

Furthermore, it was acknowledged that the agenda is so enormous that there were inevitably decisions made that many senior/middle managers were not involved in themselves – often decisions were taken at an executive level, at closed board meetings. In other words, it was not only users who found them-selves excluded from the decision-making process at times, but also some professionals and managers. This confusion was not restricted to health-service managers but is part of the confusion in the user movement in general where, as Beresford and Harding have pointed out, there are two main models in people's minds, namely 'comment' and 'control'. The first is service-centred and the second people-centred (Beresford and Harding 1993).

Health needs assessment

Within this context, in our fieldwork areas, there was evidence of serious attempts to involve users in HNA, particularly in the early days following the publication of *Local Voices*. The difficulties and problems associated with this are not small. While the goal of HNA is to 'support decision making by recom-mending options based on information about health problems, health re-sources and health outcomes in order to target resource distribution to improve health' (Area 1, Health Needs Assessment policy document), out-comes remain extremely difficult to quantify in community health services, so option appraisal is problematic. Even where options can be assessed, choice is limited by the existence of provider units offering very particular services. As a result, as one public health consultant explained:

> 'There is a tendency . . . to define the needs in terms of what is available. I have to be very careful that I'm defining the needs not just in terms of what's available, but in terms of what's potentially available.'

Purchaser planners in Area 1 claimed to be working assiduously at how services could be linked to identified needs. However they recognized that the process could indeed be lengthy: 'it might be a year . . . it might actually be five or ten years' before that point is reached (public health consultant, Area 1). Within these necessarily constricted parameters, however, there was evidence of willingness among purchasers to involve users in the process of assessing needs. In Area 2, a 'local voices' programme was developed in 1993 on the premise that some action would be taken as a result of consultation. It in-cluded user perspectives in HNA for maternity and mental health strategies, family planning and teenage sexual health. Additionally, in cooperation with the provider, there were developments in community health assessment and quality issues, including the setting up of user forums.

The purchasing authority in Area 1 likewise established several project teams also involving users, looking at different target groups for HNA – elderly people, alcohol misuse, mental health, sexual health, healthy pregnancy and infancy. Area 3 also developed a strategic approach to needs assessment, with health-strategy managers focusing on client groups including children, old people and carers. Working closely with these client groups, and the primary health-care team, it was hoped that their partially met or unmet needs would then be fed directly into the contracting process to be translated into service specifications as block contracts (see p. 11) were replaced by more sensitive instruments.

By mid-1995, however, users tended to be focused around specific issues and were drawn into the contracting process on an ad hoc basis, as issues arose, though there were plans to tie them into the process of developing health policy in a more consistent manner. One purchasing officer remained sceptical, however, about the rigour with which public health consultants were inclined to draw in users. As she observed:

'At the moment, there's whatever health needs assessment people feel like doing – which may or may not involve users, depending on what people feel like. So consequently, any service specs written from Health Needs Assessment may or may not have user involvement and some service specs are written without any reference to HNA, which may or may not have had any user influence and because we don't plan properly, we'll involve users when it suits us and generally not when it suits them.'

Nevertheless, although ad hoc and focusing on specific issues, where users did have input into explicit policy formulation there were some obvious successes. For example, in Area 1, for mental health crisis care in 1993 there was a direct link between recommendations of a local users' group and services, namely a 24-hour helpline. Also, in the field of eye care, an expressed need for help in strategies for daily living resulted in the health authority contracting with social services for a rehabilitation officer. In Area 2 a 'Health Shop' (Young Person's Family Planning Centre) was established as a direct result of focus groups which took place with the public health consultant.

After an initial period of enthusiasm, however, increasing disillusionment was apparent among managers in all three areas concerning the degree to which it was possible to involve users in HNA. Some friction was evident between purchasers and providers over the issue of HNA. According to a purchaser planner in Area 1, providers had not been particularly interested in altering the services they provide in order to meet needs ('So many of them are in a monopoly position and so medically dominated, that they are not interested'), although this was less so with community providers compared with acute providers. Large-scale consultations took place around the maternity and changing childbirth agenda, children's services, primary care resource centres and hospital closures. Health needs assessment was considered to have been subsumed in that 'that's health needs assessment in a way,' as one manager explained. These initiatives were isolated and did not involve a continuing relationship with communities or client/service groups.

In general, there was very little possibility for local views to determine the HNAs which were undertaken. Instead, they were mainly a result of national and regional directives which left little time and few resources for evaluating local needs. This was not necessarily a bad thing in the view of certain managers. A planning officer in Area 2 believed strongly that the HNA exercises that had been undertaken in that area were arbitrary – often the result of the personal interest of the public health consultants involved, rather than any view of the larger picture and context.

Planning services and service specifications

Across all three areas, considerable consultation occurred over the purchasing plan. In Area 2, almost 100 voluntary groups were contacted, draft summaries were distributed to public places and advertisements appeared in local papers inviting comments, to which 90 individuals responded. However, the responses had little effect on the purchasing plan. The aim within the purchasing organization was that the information should be used as purchasing intelligence to influence the following year's plan, but this was seen as not feasible for 1996–7.

In other cases, where needs assessments produced information regarding user views, these were not necessarily implemented. For example, in consultations over alcohol services in Area 2, while it emerged from discussions that users wanted to be involved in saying what worked and in assessing the services, this was not included in the contract. Indeed, not surprisingly, given the difficulties surrounding the nature of outcome measurements, users were not involved in monitoring outcomes, nor were they involved in any quality monitoring operations, except through community health councils (CHCs), partly because purchasers appeared to consider this predominantly a provider issue.

In relation to the purchasing plan, user and voluntary groups complained that their presence in planning, where it occurred, was largely tokenism, because decisions were taken elsewhere, at more senior levels. As one user group representative described:

'You can guarantee that [when] they form any sort of forum for discussion with people at our level, not just in the voluntary sector but people at ground level, you can be sure that there is a steering committee above them.'

Comments were invited, moreover, on the broad elements of planning rather than the detail. When sent a draft of the purchasing plan of Area 2, this representative sent it back with the comment 'This isn't a plan; this is a vague statement'. Indeed, the draft purchasing plan contained general statements about which it would have been difficult to make any comment. The outline draft included statements of intent. Under 'Primary Care Nursing', for example: to develop more flexible nursing teams around local doctors' surgeries; to meet the needs of patients being cared for in the community and those discharged from hospital. In terms of inviting a response, such statements are so vague as to be more or less meaningless other than in terms of a statement of goodwill.

As one user group representative commented:

'We've had various things through the post about them (purchasing plans, etc.) but it's all totally indistinct and vague; it means nothing. They're just general statements about broad intentions; they don't actually mean anything.'

Doubt was expressed by some voluntary group representatives, moreover, about the significance of a purchasing plan altogether. Service planning was dismissed by one group as a 'waste of time' as, they claimed, 'planning is a political process; it's about power and control, not about "rational" planning'.

Scepticism was also expressed about the purchasing plan's capacity to effect change. In terms of its financial allocations and its ability to break up block contracts, it was applauded as worthwhile, but otherwise: 'It doesn't have much effect – working on the ground and with particular managers and trying to change things is much more effective than getting involved in the purchasing plan.'

Involvement with specific issues or client groups can also have less effect than managers and professionals may wish. As the chief officer of a voluntary group in one area commented: 'Health authority/Trust managers have pet projects which get inflated, which they talk about a lot and which they're proud of, but which aren't as meaningful as they make out'. Whether involvement was centred on purchasing plans or more specific issues, user groups complained generally about the lack of feedback. Of a rapid appraisal exercise carried out jointly by social services and the health authority, one voluntary group representative commented: 'The results were just shut away in a cupboard and completely different things were carried out.'

Further, revisions did not necessarily take place as a result of user involvement. Sometimes this was not even built into the timescale of the contractual cycle, and this gave rise to considerable scepticism. According to the purchasing manager of Area 2, 'Whether it will be to seek users' views to influence the options, or whether it will be to seek user views once a series of options has been established, remains to be decided.'

In their internal appraisals of the purchasing plan consultations, moreover, purchaser managers within Area 2 acknowledged many of these failings. Reviewing the purchasing plan consultations of the 1994–5 purchasing plan, they noted some positive aspects, which included the fact that they had acknowledged the limitations inherent in the consultation process, informing users of the likely constraints to their ability to respond to comments and the difficulties in actually making change. However, the timescale allotted for the consultation was acknowledged to be too short and, more importantly, it was recognised that no organized public response was made to the public's views in the aftermath and that this had generated a good deal of public mistrust. The 1995–6 purchasing plan consultation was, in the terms of their own appraisal, beset with similar difficulties and the Area 2 CHCs' response to this consultation urged: 'the Health Authority . . . need to demonstrate positively that they not only listen to local voices, but act upon what people say'.

In the 1994–5 purchasing plan consultations, a number of specific service changes were proposed in Area 2. As a result of these comments, an internal draft circulated within the purchasing body which recommended, among other things: more investment in acute mental health care, in hospital or community settings; in maternity services, the agreeing of a process for developing service specifications that draw on studies of women's views and reflect their needs and wishes; and work with providers to introduce ethnic monitoring and establish sound information to help develop services. Significantly, none of these was explicitly expressed in the final contracts.

The comments elicited in the 1995–6 purchasing plan consultations resulted in an internal document recommending (among other things) the following actions in contracts with providers: user involvement in planning and management of mental health services and services for older people; services' accessibility to disabled people; and in maternity services, the setting of targets for continuity of care. It was far from clear whether these measures were incorporated in final contract documentation. However, one contract dealing with mental health and care in the community for elderly people, did reflect some of these concerns:

> The Trust will involve users in the planning and development of services. They will provide the Health Commission, by September 1995, with evidence of regular meetings between clinical directorates, managers of services, and service users.

Purchaser–provider relations and local voices

Although local voices is a purchaser-led strategy, as we noted earlier, the boundaries between purchasers and providers in dealing with local views can sometimes become blurred. Our data indicate that the needs of service users were being taken more into consideration by providers as they attempt to market their services across locality boundaries. For example, a provider trust in Area 1 considered ways of involving people in the business-planning process. This was seen as increasing the marketability of the Trust, although this was not their principal concern. As the service development manager explained: 'We could use it as a tool to develop innovative services. We can then make them marketable. But we have to build a collaborative relationship, we can't use it against the purchaser.'

The main consideration of the provider, therefore, was not the user but the purchaser. As one provider manager expressed it: 'We tie needs to our skills and then market and sell this to the purchaser.' Purchaser–provider relationships in our fieldwork localities were sometimes conflictual and this had effects on various aspects of the commissioning process, including the manner in which local people were incorporated into the process.

There were very few attempts by providers to involve users directly in the planning of services. For example, within one community Trust, an attempt to involve users more closely in service planning experienced a lot of opposition. In Area 1, a user–carer participation strategy was devised by the service development manager, with the aim of elderly people within that particular locality being responsible for writing their own health-care strategy. This was rejected by the Trust board, however, who felt that users would not have sufficient knowledge and training. This was then put forward to the local authority/DHA committee in an amended form, so that a project worker would work with the elderly people in assisting them in this process. This was also rejected. A more limited view of user participation was acceptable, however, with users taking part in focus groups and surveys around clinical audit projects in chiropody, audiology and physiotherapy.

By the end of 1994, patient satisfaction questionnaires were beginning to be sent on to the purchaser by providers, not, in some cases, without a degree of reluctance, despite this being built into the contracts. For example, in Area 2, by December 1994 one local Trust had agreed to produce an annual report on their surveys of users of services. Another Trust had carried out surveys as part of a value for money study. However, a third Trust claimed nothing to report and, indeed, had been unwilling to cooperate with the CHC's surveys. This record of achievement was meagre, when it is compared with the check-list of Area 2 with regard to working with the provider, which included: discovering whether user views of services were obtained as part of a planned programme that covers all services; what skills/expertise are in place for obtaining user views; by what means user views are currently obtained; whether any new internal quality standards had been set as a result of obtaining user views; examples of changes to services made as a result of obtaining user views.

Priority setting

Priority-setting exercises, involving users, occurred in various ways in our fieldwork areas. In Area 1, a priority search was undertaken in 1992, using rapid appraisal methodology, and the most important concerns high-lighted through that exercise concerned emergency services, which were tackled through contracting. In Area 2, similarly, a purchaser group met on a regular basis to consider priorities for health care in the centre of the city, while priority setting also took place in the context of the major locality project undertaken in that area. However, among managers in all three areas, there was general agreement that priority-setting by users would not be useful and might even indeed prove harmful in terms of overall pri-orities and equity issues – they were most useful in terms of acting as reference groups. As one senior purchasing manager in Area 2 explained, he did not wish to see his organization adopting the 'Oregon' approach because:

> 'I'm not convinced that consulting the public about what the priorities for health care is . . . the right thing to do . . . services like HIV/AIDS, alcohol, etc., will not get a high rating [and consequently such services will be withdrawn] so . . . while in principle I think we should be reflect-ing the views of the public, if the implications are that, then I'm not prepared to go there because I do not believe that is in the best interests of the public.'

This potential clash between ordinary citizens and professionals in priority ranking was similarly observed in a study in Inner London (see Bowling *et al.* 1993).

Users' views: the problem of diversity

We have already discussed the varied nature of user and voluntary groups that exist, and the constitution of these groups and their relationship to the health-care system is complex. Voluntary groups set up to deal with a particular issue are not necessarily representative of the relevant universe or population of users whom they could theoretically be seen to represent and user groups and carer groups operating in the voluntary sector may represent quite different sorts of interests in relation to the same health need or health-service issue. Voluntary groups are geared up to inform managers and professionals more about service gaps or service experience, knowledgeable as they are about the workings of the health service. Contact with the more general population of users is, understandably, considerably lower than contact with voluntary groups for both methodological and 'political' reasons. As one informant, herself wholly committed to the idea of incorporating user involvement into the planning process, explained, 'I've only ever been in touch with users through the post'.

Within the fieldwork areas certain user and voluntary groups appeared to predominate in the sense of being more visible and involved with consultations. There were various reasons for this. Some predominated because national priorities hinged around their client group, and this applied to groups in the mental health, carers and childbirth fields most obviously. In other cases, groups may not have felt confident enough to engage in meetings with the health commission if they lacked experience in translating their personal experiences into public issues. Those who did make this transition were inevitably, to some extent, self-selected, and this could lead to their being dismissed as 'unrepresentative'. As one purchaser manager suggested, 'those who shout loudest get their voices heard'. Applying the same logic, user representatives were able to argue that purchasers were self-selective in whom they consulted over particular issues. As one voluntary group representative said scornfully: 'They're trying to close a service down in one area and they are talking to users [from another part of town] which is totally out of order. They choose and pick who they want to consult.' Another user representative suggested:

> 'There's no formality about it; it's totally informal. People pick and choose, they talk to people they know, people they can get on with . . . they placate people, and they play one person off against another.'

This difficulty of developing established networks with local people for the purposes of consultation was not helped by the major reorganizations of departments and personnel in the purchaser organizations. However, the fluidity and unsettled nature of the market did mean that informal networks could be exploited fruitfully, with certain individuals having regular telephone contact with chief executives: 'I can if I want [pick up the phone and] say, "I'd like to talk to you".' For others the ad hoc nature and informality of the system could be less than helpful. A member of a self-help group for disabled people explained how they often received notifications of meetings with only a day's notice – insufficient for a disabled person to make the necessary arrangements for getting to the meeting. In addition, professionalism and officialdom was

often perceived to intrude, with health and social care managers hiding behind their titles and status: 'It's very daunting, you've still got them walking in
their "white coats" [saying] "I'm the chief executive of what-have-you".'

Levels of involvement

It is well understood that there are degrees of involvement – rungs on a 'ladder
of participation' (Arnstein 1969). As we have seen, purchasing authorities in
our fieldwork areas made several attempts to consult the carers and user groups
in their 'local voices' initiatives and locality projects. But there was a concern
among voluntary groups that their involvement in higher-level planning was
less complete than it might be.

A workshop held in 1994 by a local voices group in Area 2 used a version of
Arnstein's ladder, and asked participants in the workshop, several of them
purchaser representatives, to locate current projects at points on the ladder.
The ladder starts from a low degree of participation and progresses to the
individual receiving information, being consulted, advising, planning jointly,
having delegated authority and having control. Blocks to higher participation
were identified by participants and these blocks included the fact that the
public lacks the ability or training to take greater control, and that health
authority planners have to be more strategic than groups of users can be,
balancing out the needs of other groups and taking matters of equity into
consideration. The 1994–5 purchasing plan, however, was rather lower on the
scale. Participants admitted: 'It's somewhere between "advises" and "plans
jointly." If we want to be harsh we'll say "is consulted".' It was acknowledged,
however, to be an improvement on the previous year's plan which was posi-
tioned at 'is consulted'.

Underlying such tokenism on the part of purchasers may be a real or imag-
ined fear of involving users, most specifically a fear of raising expectations
which they are then unable to meet. This fear may be overplayed and may be
an example of the reluctance of health authorities to give up 'control'. Moreover, as Barnes and Wistow (1992: 11–12) have suggested, once users are involved in planning and decision-making, '. . . consensus is likely to be rare and
user involvement is likely to complicate rather than simplify decision-making
about resource allocation and directions for service development'.

Purchasers and users often had different perspectives on the degree of consultation that had actually taken place. While in Area 2, informants described
their attempt to draw users into the consultation process as 'proactive consultation', a user group in the same area was less impressed: 'Being sent a
summary of the 1994–5 purchasing plan and allowed two to three weeks to
respond to it was neither adequate nor feasible.' While some organizations felt
that they had at last been recognized and accepted by the health authorities,
those who had been invited to join local planning groups sometimes felt that
important decisions were being taken elsewhere and that the results of consultations seemed to have been overlooked. There was a common suspicion
that the authorities had already made up their minds before consultation.

The role of community health councils

The role of the CHC needs to be treated separately because of the statutory role of patients' watchdog that CHCs have occupied since 1974. The introduction of the internal market has created particular dilemmas for CHCs because, with the limited resources at their disposal, they have had to develop new kinds of relationships with purchasers, providers and the voluntary organizations. There have been no official indications of a desire to extend or strengthen the role of CHCs. However, the Government's guidance has indicated the importance of CHCs being attached to the purchasing function (Department of Health 1992; NHS Management Executive 1994) and in the policy statement on 'local voices' it is suggested of CHCs that: 'their independence can facilitate dialogue with local people and provide a valuable means to understand local views' (NHS Management Executive 1992: 6).

Since the statutory powers given to CHCs do not go far enough to facilitate their new operational role, they have to negotiate their own means of dealing with the players in the reformed system, relying on more informal channels of influence. As one CHC chief officer stated:

> 'A lot of it now with successful CHCs is about trying to develop involvement rather than consultation, trying to develop influence rather than relying on regulations and statutes, trying to persuade rather than fight. That's much more dependent on people's attitudes than anything written down.'

The viability of the CHC as a representative of people's views has also been rendered more ambiguous by the development of health authorities themselves as so-called 'champions of the people'. As the FHSA manager in Area 2 put it: '. . . in an ideal world the CHCs would become redundant because we'd have an arm of our organization called "Consumer Affairs" or whatever, which would be respected as the voice of the people'. Moreover, as the chair of the Area 2 CHC suggested: 'There is a danger of the CHCs becoming external agents of the health authority *and* being themselves mistaken for "Local Voices".'

As we have indicated, however, the extent to which the purchasers were 'in touch' with local people was often questioned, and providers often present themselves as being much more closely involved since it is they who are engaged in hands-on care. One CHC had succeeded in negotiating a statement of cooperation with each of the local providers also, the general attitude being summed up in the words of the chief officer as follows: 'My approach is to first of all try to influence the purchaser about what they buy and how they buy it and then go to the provider and try and influence how they provide it' – a kind of balancing act which effectively involves playing one off against the other. The chief officer felt that the CHC's input was very valuable for the reason that they picked up a lot more information than the purchasers do, most of whom do not live in the locality whose health needs they serve.

Obstacles to user involvement in planning health care

In spite of expressed willingness to involve local people as users and potential users in various aspects of the commissioning and decision-making process, a number of obstacles make this difficult. A fundamental tension lies in responding to need in the context of resource constraints. To this extent, there is a tension between the 'market model' which entails increasing choice and ostensible user empowerment and the 'bureaucratic model' which comprises strict rationing and equitable distribution combined with fair distribution on the basis of frozen budgets and rising demand. Where needs and resources conflict, needs are likely to go by the wayside.

As previously indicated, differences in the power and social status of users as compared with service providers mean that users may not have a powerful position in the negotiating process. In our fieldwork areas, there was some concern among purchasers that local people may be used to suit a particular agenda, and otherwise disregarded. As one purchasing officer believed:

> 'I think this organization uses the users or the voluntary sector, and you have to be constantly guarding against that . . . look at the way the [particular local] consultation is going – it's driven by the need to get answers from users for certain questions and apart from that it doesn't really matter too much.'

One of the other difficulties was potential friction between the needs of users and those of carers. While carers are often service users in their own right, those identified as carers must not be expected to speak for whom they provide support (Morris 1994). This was a constant refrain throughout the process of user involvement, where proxies and representatives are often substituted for users.

A further problem was inadequate information, because accurate information systems are lacking for purchaser, provider and user alike. Means *et al.* (1994) see this as a major difficulty in the successful implementation of the quasi-market system where the purchaser selects a provider of low quality as a result of unreliable and inaccurate information sources. This, too, diminishes the prospect of user choice. Even where the choice exists, ordinary people often lack the knowledge to distinguish between different kinds of services, especially where this may involve technology. This is very obvious in the relationship with the GP, for example, where the patient's relationship with the GP is overwhelmingly one of dependency, preventing him or her from acting as a 'good consumer' (Shackley and Ryan 1994). As Pilgrim and Rogers (1993: 166) point out:

> Doubts exist as to whether users of health services are currently in a position to make informed choices.

Thus, in our fieldwork areas, several real obstacles can be identified as getting in the way of involving users. First, the lack of planning in the organization made it difficult to integrate user involvement effectively. Secondly, purchasers were concerned that too detailed a process of user involvement would produce information that they did not want or could not use. Thirdly, those people who did respond to questionnaires or participate in public meetings were suspected of not fully representing opinion in the population as a whole. Fourthly, there was concern about the raising of expectations in a context of insufficient resources. Fifthly, purchasers felt that users and other local people did not appreciate that their views were only one perspective to be taken into account in the purchasing process, and that not acting on users' views could wrongly be taken as evidence that they were not being listened to. Finally, many of our fieldwork areas were scenes of considerable organizational instability, and this made continuity difficult to sustain across the different phases of the purchasing process. In such situations, the question of how to facilitate user involvement was not necessarily uppermost in commissioners' minds.

Organizational change and the purchaser–provider split had led to seemingly haphazard contacts with voluntary and user organizations. This situation confused users and voluntary groups. One voluntary group representative could still comment, in the summer of 1994: 'I get totally confused over purchaser and provider. I'm lost in the system, I think most people are.' Another complained, 'How on earth are you supposed to build up a relationship? . . . Every time you phone up it's a different person,' referring to the constant changing of personnel from their posts. As a result, it appeared to these groups that the onus was upon them to make contact with health and social care personnel, rather than the other way round, and to some this indeed constituted a barrier.

Conclusion

In this chapter, we have looked at the extent to which the claims of listening to local voices have been fulfilled in local policy and practice within three health authority localities. Using data collected with purchasers, providers and users, we have examined the role of local people with respect to HNA and other aspects of the commissioning cycle. Our analysis indicates considerable willingness to involve local people, but also major uncertainties as to how this should be achieved in practical terms, and what implications it might have for the commissioning and contracting process, and indeed, what the ultimate purpose should be.

We have noted several possible restrictions on involving local users: difficulties in specifying outcomes in contracts, uncertainty about how to build local voices information into purchasing plans and the continuation of block contracts which lack flexibility and sensitivity to the needs and preferences of users. Purchasers are limited by what is actually offered by the CHS Trusts and also by fear of raising expectations among users which they may then be unable to meet. Poor planning within the organization, itself partly the result of organizational turbulence, makes it difficult to involve users at a time when their input would be effective. This is combined with reluctance to take on board fully what users believe to be salient issues. Lay voices are only one part of a three-part equation in decision-making, which must include professional and clinical views as well.

One might ask if contracts have had any effect on user involvement, whether positive or negative. Opinion among health-service professionals was not particularly strong on this point. As one provider manager explained, there was very little user involvement before contracts, so it would be impossible to see anything negative about contracts. A purchaser officer felt that contracts potentially would be an excellent way of involving users, but they need to be more imaginatively constructed, in order to appeal to user interest. However, the idea of contracting is often viewed as an end in its own right, rather than the culmination of earlier phases, in which users' views would perhaps play more of a part. As Clark *et al.* (1995: 1201) comment: 'In the tendency to focus on contracting as the dynamic and operational phase of purchasing, the initial phases of the cycle have been nudged to one side.'

A further profound difficulty was the effect of reductions in the level of resources within the case-study region. In particular, discussions between purchasers and providers were dominated more by issues of financial exigencies than by creative thinking about local voices. There is, as Donaldson (1995: 24) has argued, '. . . a long way to go before what the public wants and what the health service provides are better matched,' and that will require the development of a more open and democratic health-care system with better mechanisms for linking local voices to the policy process. Some have argued that the emergence of GP fundholding, and the extended role of GPs in health commissioning generally, might serve as another means of incorporating patients' interests in quasi-market contracting. Chapter 5 therefore considers the important role of GP fundholders (and GPs) in purchasing CHS.

5

Paradoxes of

general practitioner

fundholding

This chapter considers GP fundholders' relationship with CHS providers within the quasi-market (see Chapter 1) and also considers some of the inherent paradoxes and tensions in their purchasing role. Using qualitative data from an interview survey, it is argued that while many fundholders welcome the influence that contracting offers, they are very committed to maintaining their links with local CHS providers and place a high value on the professionalism of community nursing. Although GP fundholders expressed satisfaction with the quality of the community services provided, they also reported problems in obtaining reliable and meaningful information, criticized management costs and in face-to-face negotiations with Trusts, displayed adversarial bargaining strategies.

Quasi-market contracting in primary care has created conditions in which the much sought-after integration of the primary health-care team is potentially threatened by competition. The demands and preferences of some GP fundholder practices may contradict the wider health needs of a locality identified by a DHA and may not be easily combined with the numerous other tasks of district nurses, health visitors and community-based therapists serving not just the patients on a doctor's list but a local population. It is possible that the network structure which characterizes primary care may be fractured by the aggregate effect of individual GP fundholder purchasing decisions.

According to Duggan (1995: 64), 'broadly, primary health care can be understood as accessible, holistic, continuing and personalised, and delivered by highly trained generalists, supported by community based specialists, linked to a wider network of social care'. The boundaries between primary and community health services are necessarily indistinct and the boundaries with acute care are increasingly blurred, with continually greater use being made of hospital outreach services. However, primary health care can be further distinguished from other forms of health-care provisions in that it is expected to provide the following: the first point of contact for the individual seeking help; direct access for the individual; care for the whole person in a continuing relationship; and coordinated care, providing a gateway to a range of other services (Duggan, ibid.). Community health services are an inextricable and fundamental element in primary care. It is therefore extremely important to understand the rationales used by fundholders in their contracting for those services.

The place of general practice in the NHS

A number of specific policy initiatives have marked growing state interest in, and the wider social relevance of, general practice and GPs. Indeed, the Government's publications and initiatives relevant to primary health care include: the 1986 Green Paper on primary care; the Cumberlege Report on neighbourhood nursing and the Audit Commission's study on community care (1986); the 1987 White Paper *Promoting Better Health*; the 1989 White Paper *Working for Patients*; and the new contract for GPs, introduced in 1990. Other enquiries such as the 1988 Acheson investigation into public health medicine in the NHS, the plans for social care laid down in the 1989 White Paper *Caring for People* and the *Nursing in the Community* paper (NHS Management Executive 1990d) and its 1991 document on the investigation of primary and secondary services have fundamentally changed the context of primary health care in the UK (see Taylor 1991). In 1991, GP fundholding was introduced as the linchpin of the reforms to purchasing within the NHS internal market. By 1994, fundholders' budgets totalled about 9 per cent of NHS resources (National Audit Office 1994). In order to understand the impact of these changes on community health services, it is necessary to briefly review current discussion of the advantages and disadvantages of fundholding in general practice, and the responses of GPs to current policy initiatives, and relate such changes to the historical development of general practice within the NHS.

The *Working for Patients* White Paper (Department of Health 1989a) revealed central government's determination to take a more active role in the organization of primary care. Its aims were: to make services more responsive to the consumer; raise standards of care; promote health and prevent illness; give patients a wider range of choice in obtaining high-quality primary-care services; obtain better value for money; and set clear priorities for the family-practitioner service in relation to the rest of the health service.

There was, however, concerted opposition by the British Medical Association, both to the GP contract which emerged, and to attempts to cash-limit general practitioners, which slowed down the evolution of fund holding (see, for example, Medical Practitioners' Union 1992). Although GPs were already under contract to family health services authorities, it seemed that the reforms posed a challenge to the traditional professional dominance of GPs and opened up a possibility of more managerial control (Calnan and Gabe 1991). In fact, however, fundholding GPs have increased their power and influence over their hospital colleagues: for the first time since the establishment of the NHS, consultants now have to seek the GP fundholder's business.

Issues of professional autonomy and managerial control also affect primary and community services, in relation to the family health service authority, GP and (community) nursing interface. There is some tension between the newer 'managerial' role of the GP fundholders within the practice and primary health-care team and the closer management of GPs by the family health service authority (Audit Commission 1993).

There is also some uncertainty about the impact of contracting on the structure of, and interdependency within, the primary health-care team. Professions allied to medicine are concerned about the effects of GP fundholding on their own professions. Some observers believe that the trend is away from an integrated universal community nursing service and towards a primary health-care service in which GPs have the whip hand. For example, Robin (1992: 65) has argued that: 'Issues of child protection, public health and community needs will be obvious casualties of the system.' Health visitors also foresee the end of their autonomy ahead: once there are sufficient fundholders, it is feared that GPs will increasingly determine the nature of health visiting. This eventuality has been described as 'an extraordinary end to 150 years as a proud, independent profession' (Barker 1992: 450). Similarly, district nurses fear that their high grading (and costs) will lead to problems for their profession, when negotiating contracts with both GP fundholders and health authorities (Traynor and Wade 1994). This has implications for the development of primary health-care teams because practitioner values and practice values may sometimes conflict and give rise to tension.

Thus, with the development of the internal market, GPs have found themselves with an increasingly vital role on both sides of the purchaser–provider divide. They have a key role as providers in coordinating a health-care system based upon primary care (Williams *et al.* 1993) and they have a fundamental role as *purchasers* in stimulating the development of competitive activity within the NHS. It is the ramifications of this latter role that we focus on here. We draw upon data which emerged from semistructured interviews with a purposive sample of fundholders and non-fundholders (see Appendix for further details).

Fundholding and the purchasing of community health services

Fundholding has been implemented gradually, with the requirements for practices wishing to apply for fundholding status being modified and the powers of fundholding being extended in stages. It was introduced in April 1991, when practices with more than 9000 patients could apply to join the scheme. The budget covered hospital inpatient care for a restricted range of operations, all outpatient visits, diagnostic tests done on an outpatient basis, pharmaceuticals prescribed by the practice and practice staff. Fundholders had no choice over CHS and had to contract for all the community services from an existing health service community unit.

The fundholding scheme was extended in April 1993 to include CHS for the first time, including district nursing, health visiting, chiropody, dietetics, all community and outpatient mental health services, mental health counselling, and health services for people with learning disabilities. The Department of Health ruled that practices could only purchase from established NHS community units, i.e. GPs would not be allowed to employ community staff directly or through the private sector. The form of the contract was also limited in so far as GPs could only use fixed-price, non-attributable contracts. These would not be sensitive to volume or activity levels and would not identify the costs of individual patients. These restrictions continued until 1994–5.

In 1995, the fundholding scheme was extended to incorporate more GPs and to increase the range of services covered. The dominant theme is a 'primary care-led NHS' in which purchasing decisions are taken as close as possible to the patients. From April 1995, family health service authorities and district health authorities were merged into new single authorities, to develop integrated strategies for meeting needs across primary and secondary care boundaries.

At the same time, three types of GP fundholding were introduced (NHS Executive 1994b):

- Community fundholding for small practices (up to about 3000 patients) which enables GP fundholders to buy most community health services (but this excludes all acute hospital treatments).
- Standard fundholding (for practices with over 5000 patients) which includes most elective surgery and outpatient work, specialist nursing and CHS.
- Total purchasing (in a small number of pilot projects) where GPs can purchase all hospital and community services.

In the case-study areas, in all the Trusts there was some anxiety about 'competition', and providers all expressed concern about winning business from fundholders. However, this was not always endorsed by all CHS staff. For example, in one community Trust, at a marketing seminar held for professional heads of services, there was a general level of scepticism about the potential importance of fundholders. As one service head remarked: 'We've only got eight GP fundholders – why spend a lot marketing services to them?' Nevertheless, the managers of each Trust in the three areas were extremely concerned about securing and increasing GP fundholder income and encouraged their staff accordingly.

In fact, there is a paradox with regard to the perception of fundholders as customers who are difficult to secure. On the one hand, providers perceived GP fundholders as much more volatile than large DHA purchasers who are less likely to move to other providers and start building relationships with new provider agencies. But the organizational problems of size and unwieldy infrastructure do not exist for GPs who had already been willing to change acute providers at the end of the contract period. On the other hand, there was a cultural perception that GP fundholders' personal knowledge of, and well-established links with, individual CHS professionals are of more importance to fundholders than to DHAs or commissions, and this encouraged loyalty on the part of GPs.

The study by Glennerster *et al.* (1994) noted that in acute services, GPs have had the motivation and the information to seek better contracts. They have switched to more effective providers, or have improved the performance of the same provider. This choice, however, has not been available for the purchasing of community health services. They point out that the nature of purchasing by fundholders of community health services and the considerable limitations that have existed, have led to GPs complaining that giving them a budget in these circumstances was a fiction, because their freedom was nothing like as great as with hospital services. The analogy of 'customers going to another shop' does not really apply to the pattern of GP purchasing of community health services, firstly because of the value placed on professional and personal loyalties and also because the problems of information in CHS (as shown earlier) make it extremely difficult to compare services being offered by other Trusts with the services currently being received. In other words, monitoring difficulties place even more significance on these networks of professional trust.

Broadly, our data confirm these findings. Interviews with GP fundholders (and non-fundholding GPs) revealed beliefs and actions consistent with the argument outlined in Chapter 1, viz. that CHS, by definition, exhibit many of the characteristics which make network structures and 'clan' forms of organization inevitable. That is, networks, partnerships and trust are intrinsic to their operation, and the kind of contracting which develops from this must be relational rather than adversarial in approach. However, there were also indications that some GP fundholders did invoke *competitive* arguments to legitimate their demands and from fieldwork observation (and some interviews) a few behaved in an adversarial way in contract negotiations with providers. These views are supported by qualitative data concerning fundholders' purchasing behaviour with regard to CHS.

We will now examine the relationship between these parties including: reasons why GPs choose to go fundholding; GP fundholders' relationship with community health service professionals and the primary health-care team; relationships with provider Trusts; the results of contracting for CHS; and attitudes towards fundholding held by non-fundholders.

Why do GPs choose to go fundholding?

The two issues upon which fundholding revolve can be summarized as choice and control. All respondents subscribed to the view that going fundholding meant a better service for patients and a greatly increased opportunity to influence patient care. GP fundholders were largely interested in changing the nature of *acute* services, especially in orthopaedics, dermatology and ophthalmology, and all claimed to have been successful in these areas. As one prospective fundholder commented: 'Somebody with cataracts, or needs a hip replacement. What I can say to them is, "I'm on your side. It's the two of us against the system".'

In general, they were satisfied at last to be able to influence the provider units over the quality of the services they were delivering. One fundholder described the process of fundholding as a 'pump priming thing' to push hospitals into changing the services they provide. Most importantly, the improvements cited were all in the field of *acute*, rather than community, services. First- and second-wave fundholders in particular seized the opportunity to challenge old patterns and explore new possibilities. One first-wave fundholder described fundholding as a 'pathfinder activity' – all the advantages would be to push forward the boundaries of quality in care. To this degree, the fundholding system was seen as benefiting all patients, not just the patients of fundholders. A fourth-wave fundholder did not wish to be left behind, having seen the advantages accrued by fundholders: 'I was very nervous about being left out. I'd become a second-class practice.'

Most acknowledged that a two-tier system was developing but did not see their action in going fundholding as responsible for bringing this about. As one GP put it, 'there's been a two-tier system for donkey's years'. Recognizing this, they did not want to put their patients on the second tier. Yet, this recognition was balanced out by a certainty that *urgent* cases would be dealt with within the NHS where necessary so that people in real need will get the service they require. The element of choice was restricted to cases of lesser urgency. That patients of fundholders would be at an advantage over patients of non-fundholders was openly acknowledged, although the knock-on effect of an improvement of services brought about generally was considered to be of long-term advantage to both kinds of patients. Nevertheless, there was an agreement that since there was a limited pot of money, if every GP was a fundholder, then these advantages would disappear.

Reductions in hospital consultants' power was an aspect of GP fundholding welcomed by the fundholders. They saw themselves as better placed to make the decisions and decide on the priorities formerly made by the consultants. GP fundholders were willing to be involved in the rationing process and expected to develop an internal waiting list within their practices. They felt that their actions had shaken up the NHS providers and resulted in improvements within the NHS. In part, this is setting their own priorities, as opposed to acquiescing in those laid down by the consultants. The reasons prompting GPs to become fundholders thus compare very closely with the reasons given by GP fundholders in the study by Glennerster *et al.* (1992).

Attitudes towards the primary health-care team

Doctors expressed strong commitment to the population in the immediate locality and to their local primary health-care team. They placed a high degree of trust in primary health-care team relationships. Their present local CHS Trusts were preferred, provided that the quality of their services was deemed to be satisfactory – which in every case it was. Indeed, although the concept of 'quality' is nebulous in CHS, *all* the fundholders stressed that they were generally satisfied with service quality.

The source of any dissatisfaction lay rather with quantity, and the fact that the service, good as it was, was inadequate to cope with the level of demand. None of the fundholders in the study had any desire to abandon or reject the local unit. Rather, they wanted to keep it viable, while encouraging it to improve: 'contracting with responsibility' as one GP put it. While they were willing to make competitive choices in what they described as fringe services, such as physiotherapy, psychotherapy, counselling and speech therapy, this was never taken too far. 'At the end of the day, if the morale down there is bad among the staff, then that can lead to bad care for patients,' as one fundholder put it.

Fewer changes were likely to be instituted with CHS as opposed to acute services, because there was general agreement that those services needed a *locally*-based provider. As one doctor observed, 'One always considers the options, looks at it, evaluates it. But community services, by their nature, are basically area-based aren't they? I think it would be silly to get another provider to come in.' Ultimately, GPs' and GP fundholders' loyalties lay with the primary health-care team, and the CHS professionals involved, although doctors were less supportive of 'the management' situated in the Trusts.

This raises the issue about community nurses being directly employed by GPs and GP fundholders rather than being contracted through a Trust. It also relates to the fear expressed by professional nursing bodies regarding the consequences of the GP contract for their professional autonomy. According to the Medical Practitioners' Union (1992: 5–6): 'These other professional groups are no longer content to be handmaidens to doctors and are demanding their own professional autonomy and dignity . . .'

Direct employment of CHS staff, although enthusiastically talked about in the early days of fundholding, was *not* a desired aim by the GP fundholders (or GPs) in our sample. Alongside the practical difficulties it would entail, including ensuring emergency cover and cover for sick leave, were broader considerations, such as the recognized need for continuing professional development. A few fundholders claimed that they might wish to employ district nurses and health visitors directly in the future, so that these professionals would then work to their directions. But most did not see it as serving their purpose any better.

Relationship with CHS providers

The relationship with provider Trusts must be placed in the context of the acknowledged importance of local relationships noted earlier, together with the general satisfaction felt with the quality of services provided. Where alternative providers were used by GP fundholders and GPs in our sample, this was for pragmatic reasons connected with serving patients who lived outside of the catchment area of the local provider; indeed, in only one case had this occurred.

Significantly, there had been very little overt or direct marketing of services to GP fundholders by providers and very few instances of being approached by other non-local Trusts. GP fundholders reported that they had neither actively sought out information about alternative providers, nor had they been actively targeted themselves, with exceptions only occurring where GP fundholders were situated on geographical borders and had patients who lived within the catchment areas of other providers. Other approaches appear to have been very low key, with limited information sent through the post; 'Just, "We're here, and a tariff if you're interested",' as one GP fundholder described. In other words, this acknowledgement of the intrinsic nature of long-term working relationships being at the heart of contracting for CHS was to a large extent recognized on both sides.

On some occasions there were seemingly adversarial or even confrontational attitudes expressed by GP fundholders in contract negotiation meetings with Trust managers. However, these sat uneasily with the claims made in interviews that they were satisfied with the services they were receiving. In meetings with providers, some doctors explicitly asked and commented: 'What part of your strategy is for GP fundholders in particular?'; 'What are you going to do for us as your best customer?'; 'If you don't provide what we want, we will go to X or somewhere else.' This elicited conciliatory responses by the Trusts such as 'Anything the fundholders want, we'll move heaven and earth to provide'; 'We are doing quite a lot of intensive work with GP fundholders. They are requiring things and so we are adapting to meet demands.'

It thus appears that while the contracting system and the experience of bargaining and negotiation seems to permit or even encourage adversarial (and occasionally confrontational) modes of relating to each other, underlying this both parties agreed on the priority of maintaining local relationships with CHS. In practice, the value of preserving local networks was recognized as having a greater priority by GP fundholders than exploiting the possibilities open to them in a quasi-competitive market. Thus, the model favoured by GP fundholders as purchasers is that of limited contestability – the threat of moving a contract to a different supplier – rather than 'free-market' or price-oriented competition.

At the same time, GP fundholders described experiencing some frustration in their relationship with providers. This centred on the paucity of patient-based information available (generally considered to be an intrinsic problem in CHS, as noted previously) and their resulting inability to accurately monitor services. In other words, the nature of CHS as a kind of product militates against the possibility of comparing services offered by different providers and hence renders the cultivation of trust relationships essential. Most contracts in fact included arrangements about the routine reporting of information on activity (e.g. numbers of patient contacts, staff time), quality indicators (e.g. waiting time for referral) and finance (expenditure/invoicing). But while fundholders were questioned about arrangements for obtaining information and their satisfaction with procedures for monitoring the contract, none of them expressed satisfaction with this. The absence or inadequacy of information was the main concern for all respondents and was frequently referred to in reply to other questions in the interview. Indeed, as one fund manager pointed out, problems in defining precise levels of activity were a major reason why they had accepted a block contract (see p. 11), which did not require very sophisticated monitoring. She remarked: 'I don't know whether we're benefiting or they're [the Trust] benefiting really. In effect, it's not really a contract from a money point of view.'

Costs and prices elicited different responses. As one fundholder commented: 'I think the feeling is that we don't really know what we're getting for our money.' The bulk of district nursing and health visiting services were in block contracts and room for negotiation on prices charged by providers was therefore limited to the specialist therapy services, but fundholders were concerned about prices. For example, one doctor regarded the pricing of health visiting and district nursing as a 'stitch-up' because the practice's budget allocation was based on regional estimates of previous activity levels which were now outdated and there was no room for negotiation.

Despite this frustration, however, it was acknowledged that price was *not* a hugely important factor in decisions about community contracts. On the contrary, as one fundholder explained: 'There would be a lot of other factors – team building, continuity and experienced members of staff would be very high on the list. The staff . . . are really appreciated. If the standard of the service went down, then we'd be looking somewhere else I suppose.'

Generally the fundholders' relationship with providers was thought to have improved directly as a result of fundholding. All respondents replied that there had been significant changes, although they varied in identifying the type and impact of changes. One fundholder said that he now had 'more say' in how the services were provided: the Trust was 'more responsive' and had been more helpful than the local acute hospital Trust. One fundholder observed that the services themselves had broadly stayed the same but there were some new services and she was getting more feedback from the community staff: there was now a much better flow and exchange of information between professionals. Another doctor pointed out that the provider 'will listen to us, do what we want when they can'; he gave the example of providing practice-based physiotherapy which had not been possible before fundholding. Indeed, several fundholders identified the most important advantages in fundholding as having the staff on the premises, with services being carried out inhouse rather than going to the health authority clinic, 'Something that we've been aiming at for about twenty-five years, but never succeeded,' as one fundholder explained. Another fundholder said that now health visitors would visit patients living across the district boundary, but also that as a result of fundholding, community staff were more responsive to the practice's needs. He gave as an example the agreement secured for a district nurse to go on a specialist course in order to do new clinical procedures. Previously this was unlikely: 'These were things all smothered in red tape before and it's suddenly vanished.'

As we have indicated previously, CHS Trusts are fearful of losing GP fundholder business. However, while fundholders may occasionally threaten to move contracts to other providers, at the same time they value the loyalty and trust embedded in established relationships with professionals.

Undoubtedly there was some anxiety among providers about the development of GP fundholder practice-based activities. This is a different kind of threat from that provided by DHA purchasers (and acute hospital outreach services) who may ultimately question the very existence of CHS Trusts. Fundholders may wish to develop their own comprehensive service in the future so that, as one provider manager predicted: 'Unless we are prepared to provide the services the way they want we stand to lose them. I think we have to be responsive to what they want and have to be able to provide it in the environment that they want to actually maintain that business.'

The results of GP fundholders' contracting for CHS

Control over their own budgets, although time-consuming and costly in administrative and transaction terms, provides GP fundholders with the means to determine their own priorities and indeed to wrest power from the hands of the hospital consultants, with whom they had long been embattled. But does the holding of a contract actually make a real difference to fundholders' attitudes towards the CHS providers and the services they receive? Our data suggest that it does not create new demands, but formalizes, intensifies and channels the pre-existing interest GPs already had in the kind of services they are receiving.

In practice, the operation of purchasing by GP fundholders in CHS was limited throughout the period in which this study was undertaken, with the bulk of community nursing services being covered by 'fixed-price, non-attributable' block contracts and with only a smaller proportion of therapy and specialist services being covered by more detailed and precise forms of contract, namely cost and volume, and more rarely cost per case (see p. 12).

There is no doubt, however, that the process of contracting gives GP fundholders some power over the provider. 'I think it makes everybody more aware and it means that GPs particularly think they've got a right to ask for information, whereas before maybe they felt they hadn't,' as one fund manager explained. Similarly, for another doctor: 'You get more dialogue, more analysis, more effort on all sides to try and improve the services and look at their efficiency.'

Similarly, in the case study areas there was some direct GP fundholder involvement with the design of service specifications. In two districts, groups of fundholders met regularly to discuss common concerns and devised service specifications as a group. Fund managers were delegated to write detailed specifications to supplement and adapt those used by the health authority. As a result of this, they had discussions with provider staff and secured mutually acceptable agreements.

For fundholders, therefore, contracts did not appear to be valued because they stimulated supplier competition or large-scale shifts in services *per se*.

Rather, they were seen (and used) as vehicles through which the fundholder could articulate a demand for information and influence quality in a way they were unable to do before holding their own budget, but which had been a long-held aim. The purchasing process had intensified this interest and facilitated its achievement; as one fundholder expressed it, the fact that they were now buying services made them more concerned that they are getting what they pay for.

Fundholders were anxious to receive as much information as possible, in order to know what exactly they were getting for their money. Every provider manager interviewed reported that fundholders were very demanding in terms of their requests for information. As one provider manager complained: 'Everywhere you went the fundholders were moaning at you about no information, and wanting to know in fine detail what their nurses were doing every minute of the day.' Indeed, a typical complaint from fundholders centred on the sheer inadequacy of the information supplied to them. Clearly then, a crucial element in the fundholders' endorsement of the scheme was their increased power to force providers to supply increasingly detailed knowledge about their services.

Attitudes of non-fundholders towards GP purchasing

Attitudes among non-fundholders towards fundholding were mixed. They varied from the enthusiastic observer, who claimed she would definitely want to go fundholding if only her list size were large enough, to the GP struggling alone and viewing the prospect of added responsibilities and risks represented by fundholding as 'nightmarish', to the thriving group practice who maintained ethical and political objections to the concept. There were some GPs who saw predominantly the financial risks and feared them. Then there were others who saw no reason to change the way they operated, but acknowledged that, in time, they may be forced to go fundholding 'by the bullying of necessity'.

Among those who chose not to go fundholding, there were several core elements to their unwillingness to do so. One reason was the awareness of the increased administrative burden; several expressed the view that they came into medicine to become doctors, not administrators. There was also a generally shared opinion that if fundholding was taken to its logical conclusion and *everyone* became fundholders, then all advantages would be levelled out – no-one would be able to jump waiting lists, for example. One GP expressed the view that his opinions were registered and already held sway as a result of his involvement in health authority commissioning procedures.

Significantly, non-fundholders' views about the importance and quality of local community health services were identical to those expressed by GP fundholders. Indeed, GPs were content with the status quo and were relatively satisfied with the community services they were receiving and so envisaged no great advantages in going fundholding.

Evidently dissatisfaction with CHS was not high among either fundholders or ordinary GPs, and their attitudes towards fundholding were influenced by much more complex and deep-rooted sets of factors. Among those factors was their connection with, and influence over, DHA purchasing policies.

Relationship between the purchasing functions of GP fundholders and health authorities

In the relationship between DHAs and fundholders there is the possibility of both antagonism and collaboration. A degree of tension is inherent, because to some extent they are competitors, at least while DHAs continue to buy services on behalf of non-fundholding patients. At the same time, collaboration is not only practical, but probably inevitable, because they are fulfilling different, but complementary, roles, at different levels – one macro, the other micro. There is a potential conflict between the activities of GPs and the broader, population-based activities of health authorities as purchasers. In the 'Rubber Windmill' simulation of the NHS internal market organized by East Anglian Regional Health Authority, DHAs and fundholding GPs pursued separate and competing purchasing plans, and fundholders were also in competition with self-governing hospitals and local authorities to develop similar services (ACHEW 1991).

A working relationship can, nevertheless, be established with effort on both sides, despite the very different ways in which both purchasers work. For example, Shapiro's (1994) account from one metropolitan DHA's relationship with their fundholding GPs points out that there is usually a maturation period among fundholders, and after the first year's aggressive purchasing, a realization that coordination of planning is important. This is driven partly by financial constraints, but also by the thought that prioritization may be easier if it is shared between purchasers. However, at the same time, as collaboration comes about and GPs feel that their views are being noted and are helping to bring about change, then the incentive for practices to become fundholders diminishes.

There are other reasons why collaboration is important. Effective purchasing depends on substantial amounts of good quality and up-to-date information. Collaboration is the key to ensuring the provision of such data for informed health needs assessment. A locality model of some kind seems to be necessary for collaborative work both with fundholders and non-fundholders. Other studies have observed that collaboration and cooperation between health authorities and fundholders is essential in the quasi-market. Pollock and Majeed (1991) stress that to become effective commissioners of health services, fundholding GPs need skills in disciplines that are usually seen as the remit of public health specialists and health-service planners, such as epidemiology, needs assessment and health planning. In short, fundholders are expected to take on many of the roles of DHAs and FHSAs, but at a practice level.

In our case studies, various methods were used to establish closer links between GPs and the health authorities. In Area 1 (see Appendix) extensive efforts were made by the DHA to consult and involve local GPs in the district purchasing plan, as well as through regular meetings, 'forums' and special project teams. In Area 2, GP 'commissioning consultants' were appointed to the health authority to represent the views of all the GPs in the area, whether fundholding or non-fundholding. They had the task of visiting practices on a regular basis, canvassing views on general concerns and gathering information required by the health authority purchasers. One of the commissioning consultants (a non-fundholder) explained:

> 'One of the things that the purchasers felt they needed more information about was . . . they wanted some kind of confirmation that their priorities that they had chosen for health care were priorities that the GPs would agree with.'

In Area 3 there was an integrated DHA/FHSA 'commission' which coordinated the local purchasing strategy. Three different types of GP purchasing coexisted. First, the commission acted on behalf of all non-fundholding GPs in its purchasing and contract negotiation. Second, it consulted extensively and monitored fundholding practices closely. Third, there was a 'hybrid' fundholding group (combining very small practices) managed by the commission, but allowing for those GPs' highly localized preferences on services to be expressed in health authority negotiated contracts.

Conclusions

Fundholding, though a linchpin of the reforms, is taking place in a context of varied purchasing activity, which includes the activity of DHAs alone and DHA/FHSAs combined, GP commissioning and locality purchasing. However, despite the predictions of several observers, there is no obvious reason to assume that fundholding ultimately renders DHA purchasing redundant. DHAs, wanting to engineer a purchaser-driven NHS, require a range of skills concerned mainly with public health medicine, finance, contracting, planning, information, quality, communications and public relations. But the establishment of a purchaser-driven NHS requires collaboration between the different kinds of purchasers if they are to encourage a versatile and competitive system. Cooperation between fundholders and DHAs will be necessary if long-term DHA priorities in planning and health needs assessment for a large population are not to be subverted by the individualistic behaviour of fundholders responding to the demands of their small practice population.

In fact, our qualitative data suggest that compared with DHAs, GP fundholders displayed a greater commitment to relational contracting in their purchasing of CHS, placing a high value on local networks, trust and loyalty with regard to members of the primary health-care team. This behaviour in relation to CHS has also been observed by Glennerster and colleagues (1994), and is in contrast to the kind of behaviour of both GP fundholders and DHAs in relation to acute hospital services. Fundholders regard community health services as involving skills and expertise which must be provided locally, by professionals in whom they invest a great deal of trust. Fundholders are prepared to 'shop around', but only on the margins: the 'fringe' services, such as physiotherapy, chiropody, psychological services, as opposed to the core services which comprise nursing and health visiting. It is exactly this highly limited form of contracting which Paton (1992) predicted for the kind of quasi-market developing in health care.

The practical consequences of the reforms are currently being worked out at neighbourhood level, and the wider effects of fundholding, both within the context of primary care and for purchasing in general, cannot be predicted. The future of fundholding remains uncertain, as other kinds of purchasing, including locality purchasing, evolve alongside it. The situation is unclear, especially to GPs themselves. As one non-fundholding GP explained, the local DHA had talks with the local medical committee about devolving the budget to non-fundholding GPs but: 'What does that mean? Does that mean that they're then fundholding GPs? They say that they would like to devolve the budget to the non-fundholding GPs, but what that means to me is that either they are fundholding GPs being managed in a way which the DHA wants, or they're not. If they're not, what are they?' Meanwhile, empirical evidence on the impact of the scheme is still lacking (see Dixon and Glennerster 1995).

From the case study and interview data about CHS in the context of primary care and fundholding, therefore, paradoxes emerge which in many ways reflect the tensions found within national policy. The main paradoxes which emerge directly from our data are, firstly, that the fundholders we interviewed were confident about the satisfactory nature of the services they were purchasing from providers of CHS, despite their acknowledgement that the information on which they relied to make such judgements was poor. Secondly, while acknowledging that better information was necessary for them to be able to judge the quality of the services they were purchasing, at the same time they baulked at the idea of having to shoulder the increased management costs that this would inevitably imply. Thirdly, while recognizing that one way round this problem would be for them to employ practice-based therapy staff, together with wielding more control over district nurses and health visitors, they did not want the responsibilities that would come from direct employment of such staff. Fourthly, while in face-to-face negotiations with Trusts they appeared adversarial, behind the scenes they revealed themselves to be much more satisfied with the providers and aware of the need to maintain relationships of trust with professionals. Finally, they appeared to maintain a distinction between 'core' services, comprising nursing and 'fringe' or therapy services. While the current scheme of fixed-price, non-attributable contracts prevented them from modifying the core services, even if it were possible, the fundholders appeared to have no wish to do so.

These paradoxes demonstrate the conflict between the market and the clan model of organization. So, while the contracting framework encourages GP fundholders to take on an assertive role in purchasing, in community health services they are reluctant to destroy their long-term relationship with CHS professionals and their contracting behaviour reflects this ambiguity. However, as we shall see in Chapter 6, health authority purchasers adopt a quite different approach to the problems of contracting and trust.

6

Contracting and the

negotiation of trust

The creation of a quasi-market in the NHS required that purchasers and providers should formalize their relationship through contracts. From 1991 to 1993, the purchaser–provider split was gradually established, with the introduction of general practitioner (GP) fundholding and new larger health authorities and emergent Trusts being formed, many through amalgamations and mergers of pre-existing districts and units. The Government's policy on contracting ensured a 'steady state' so that major disruptions in services were avoided, and there was a period of stability as the new organizations learned their respective roles. After this initial period, GP fundholders and health authorities were encouraged to use their purchasing power to obtain improvements in services, and by 1993 it became evident (especially in acute hospital services) that significant changes were underway, some of which attracted public concern and political criticism (Ham 1994a). The internal market had begun to evolve, and its effect in some areas was to threaten the viability of long-established hospitals and specialties. The risk of immediate changes in the provision of community health services was much lower, mainly due to the fact that GP fundholders were initially required to retain existing suppliers and health authorities were preoccupied with acute hospital services and frequently gave CHS a lower priority in policy.

After 1993, however, GP fundholders were enabled to buy community services from other providers (though community nursing had to be bought from NHS Trusts) and DHAs began to consider means of stimulating greater competition among CHS Trusts. Government health ministers exhorted DHAs to adopt a more vigorous role in managing the market and the jargon of 'purchasing' was broadened to comprise 'commissioning'. The stress on commissioning connected purchasers with strategic goals of maximizing health gain through a variety of means including alliances with non-NHS agencies. It also emphasized the importance of accountability for effective use of resources and the need to promote contestability in the market (Stockford 1993; Curruthers *et al.* 1995; Øvretveit 1995).

In order to understand the process of contracting, and the dynamic relationships between purchasers and providers of CHS, it is necessary to have a detailed awareness of the experience of those engaged in the business of devising and negotiating contracts. Intensive qualitative research is particularly vital to gain an insight into actors' perceptions of salient issues, and to observe change over time. This chapter therefore presents and analyses findings from case studies of DHA purchasers and CHS providers in three large metropolitan districts, carried out over two contracting rounds, 1993–4 and 1994–5 (for further details of methodology, see the Appendix).

What were the principal concerns of those directly involved in purchasing and commissioning CHS? How did they approach the design of service specifications and how did this relate to their commissioning strategy? What did Trust managers hope to achieve from the contracts? What were the major issues during contract negotiations? We present evidence which answers these important questions. The format for discussion takes two key issues as the focal concern, and presents them by fieldwork locale (Areas 1, 2 and 3) in order to contextualize the findings: the description of the contracts' content and conditions (service specifications) and negotiations over price and volume (finance and resources).

Contract specification

The first issue comprises the problem of devising an agreed description of the services covered by contracts. As previous chapters have suggested, the scope or coverage of CHS is variable, and DHAs differ in the degree to which they wish to specify the precise content of services demanded.

Area 1

In Area 1, a block contract in 1992–3 maintained pre-existing services, based upon very broad descriptions of professional staffing and functions. In early 1993, the Trust director of contracting wanted to design better specifications and was keen to respond to the DHA's request to move towards more 'outcome-related' contracts. This was seen as a 'big jump' but a 'slow process', especially because it was difficult to identify outcomes clearly and because CHS were 'inadequately measurable'. This was linked to problems in monitoring quality – the Trust director of contracting thought that the purchaser was equally confused about how to measure outcomes but Trust professional staff were developing service standards which were being shared with health authorities.

Later that year the Trust director of contracting said that more specifications had been drafted by provider staff and the purchaser had not really been involved or made any constructive suggestions. By contrast, a purchaser consultant in public health (responsible for health needs assessment work) complained that service specifications from both acute hospitals and the community Trust were all 'vague' and mostly in 'old NHS-speak': that is, they were too dominated by existing service patterns and assumptions. Providers seemed unwilling or unable to think in terms of *needs*, but were locked into traditional models. Nonetheless, very detailed specifications might be counterproductive in stifling innovation among those actually providing the service.

According to the purchaser director of contracting, specifications were vitally important. He wanted to 'clarify what we are getting for our £x million. Where is it going? What do we want it to change to? What is the outcome of that intervention? It's by no means clear'. The current contract was really a service level agreement but he wanted 'sharper, more-focused' contracts linked to health needs assessment and quality monitoring. Developing specifications to achieve this would need more collaborative work with the provider.

Two months later, this process had started, with regular joint meetings to get detailed breakdowns of services, professional staff and client groups, and to work on expected outcomes. The contract specifications were, according to the purchaser, being developed jointly and would be linked with the purchasing plan's priorities. For this manager, the exercise was necessarily *collaborative*:

'I think it's a degree of ownership on both sides, on what is being delivered. I think there's a better understanding from both sides on what is expected to be achieved. You get more collaboration from the provider in doing that, rather than imposing something.'

Evidently this approach was successful, because specifications were not an issue for discussion or disagreement during the 1994 contract negotiations.

By the summer of 1994, joint talks and meetings about 'developing' specifications (including quality and outcome indicators) were proceeding. This was not expected to be accomplished quickly; indeed it was a task scheduled for continuing work over the next two years. Nevertheless, it was still seen as a cooperative venture, and the purchaser contract manager wanted to co-opt Trust professional staff:

'We want to get clinicians involved in actually contracting . . . Really it's to give them a degree of ownership in the actual documentation that they've actually participated in drawing up. It's not that the purchaser is seen to impose this specification and [say] "This is what they will do".'

The purchaser director of contracting argued for breaking up the current contract into different components, linking these with activity, finance and outcomes of intervention, but recognized that this was constrained by information problems. His frustration was still clear five months later when he observed that it was still difficult to get an accurate picture of the exact content of local community services, and he claimed that there was some confusion and vagueness even among Trust staff in their response to purchaser draft specifications.

Contract negotiations in early 1995 did not have any significant debate about specifications, as they were dominated by financial issues, although there was some argument about the practicality of the 'quality' section of the contract (discussed below). By May 1995, the purchaser director of contracting acknowledged that specifications were still very broad, but now accepted that precise detail was unnecessary and potentially damaging to their relationship with the Trust:

'If you start raising the question – "This isn't in the contract" – then you are destroying the relationship, because we're buying a *package*. We're specifying the main elements of a package: we're not specifying the nuts and bolts and the detail. If you start doing that, then you just build up a bureaucracy.'

The health authority director of performance management regarded the changes in specification as only 'around the margins'; there was no intrinsic difficulty doing the specifications, the main problem was in prioritizing them for resources. A purchaser public health consultant believed that health needs assessment work had only influenced specifications very marginally, and indirectly. Changing the way services are delivered was more to do with 'changing professional practice and mind-sets' rather than 'any sort of contract'.

There was a different perception in the Trust. The director of contracting did not think that the specifications were heavily influenced by either the DHA purchasing plan or the Trust business plan. The Trust supported more sophisticated specifications linked to outcomes, but had not yet been able to design them. This work was still regarded as joint with the purchaser, but as having come to a temporary halt. This manager, however, believed that some community services were inherently more difficult to specify; certain services such as children's services, learning disability services and condition-related services were relatively easier, but some aspects of community nursing were very difficult. Importantly, the director of contracting noted that GP fundholders wanted patient-based specifications, whereas the health authority was more concerned with population-based health needs, and this affected the way specifications were defined.

It can be concluded that in Area 1, the specification of services covered in the contract was not a source of serious dispute or conflict, that it was regarded as collaborative work in progress, but lack of detail or sophistication, and delays in formulating explicit outcomes-oriented specifications did not prevent the wider processes of commissioning and contracting from proceeding.

Area 2

In Area 2, the purchaser director of contracting started from a position that the purchasing plan objectives did not necessarily correspond with existing patterns of service, so specifications were important in getting a better fit. He thought that community services were not intrinsically difficult to specify, and were no different from acute services for contract purposes; lack of information was the key problem. A similar view was expressed by the acting chief executive who argued that the problems of devising specifications were found in both acute and community services; CHS were only relatively more difficult because of the absence of reliable measures of output and outcomes.

During contract negotiations in early 1993 (which were dominated by financial issues) there was debate about the implications of draft specifications and amendments to the current block contract. The Trust chief executive said that they could not meet all of the purchaser's stipulations, especially about quality requirements and *Patient's Charter* targets, without extra resources. Purchaser representatives replied that they could not sign a contract unless the Trust adhered to statutory regulations embodied in the specifications. The Trust finally acceded but with the proviso that they would only meet the quality specifications 'within allocated resources'.

During the summer of 1993, within the purchaser there was considerable discussion about making requirements about standards and quality more explicit in the specifications – current drafts were thought to be too vague and general. The quality manager acknowledged that it was difficult to link CHS specifications with either health needs assessment work or quality indicators. A purchaser consultant in public health did not think that CHS were more difficult to specify than acute hospital services, but he also believed that acute specifications lacked detail. Community contracts were often 'crude' and sometimes had 'spurious' detail.

This argument was partly acknowledged by Trust staff, but they criticized the DHA purchasing plan's assumptions about CHS. At an internal Trust meeting in September 1993, the chief executive observed that the purchasers 'don't understand how difficult community services are': the purchasing plan and their approach to specifications was sometimes too specific and sometimes too vague:

> 'They don't understand – they don't understand our financial constraints. It [the purchasing plan] is more like a traditional paper from an old-fashioned health authority. They need to be realistic about what *we* can achieve and what *they* can monitor. They have gone into too much detail.'

This view was expressed just when the local health authority had decided not to ratify the draft purchasing plan's proposal to shift resources away from acute hospitals into community services, leading to a severe financial crisis for the newly established CHS Trust, and precipitating a long series of arguments about how to implement cost savings. These problems were compounded by the fact that the Trust was in the process of incorporating community services previously provided by other units in the local conurbation. There were severe organizational difficulties which made even the description of services, let alone their detailed specification, exceptionally complicated and troublesome.

In the meantime, contract negotiation meetings were overwhelmingly concerned with financial matters and likely service reductions. At meetings in November 1993 and February 1994 the Trust objected to the purchaser's quality specification, claiming that they were inadequately resourced to provide the information requested. Eventually this was temporarily resolved by an agreement to do more 'joint' work to 'develop' quality specifications over the next year.

Constructing specifications was clearly a contentious issue in Area 2. According to the Trust director of contracting there was a marked contrast in the approach pursued by the health authority and that taken by GP fundholders. GP fundholders were said to have knowledge of the actual workings of community services and were flexible about specifications; by contrast, the DHA purchaser lacked a detailed appreciation of CHS but were more bureaucratic: 'They want everything and want to pin us down, be very specific.' The Trust's professional head of physiotherapy (who was very active in discussions with purchasers about draft service plans) commented that:

> '[Purchaser managers] show a lack of comprehension about what community services are, in their approach to specifications. Until there is a professional input, there won't be a mature relationship with the provider. It should be a *joint* role.'

The result of the overall contract negotiations was that there were disagreements on finance and service reductions, which were partially settled through regional health authority arbitration. This set the scene for purchaser–provider relationships during the rest of 1994 and the negotiations in 1995. One immediate effect was the establishment in mid-1994 of a regular meeting between health authority and Trust chief executives and senior managers. At its first meeting, the purchaser director of contracting emphasized that there was a feeling within the health authority that they did not know what they were getting for their £x million contract: 'With other Trusts we have a feeling of what we're getting, but not with community.' In reply, Trust managers stressed again the problems caused by amalgamations of services and the lack of integrated information systems, but agreed a schedule of work to identify what additional information could be supplied. Joint purchaser–provider working groups were set up to collate information about activity, finance and quality.

Subsequent meetings of the senior managers' group were mainly concerned with continued disputes about finance and the management of service reductions. However, in November 1994, the purchasers informed the Trust that they wanted to 'unpack' the current block contract into smaller contracts for specific services. The health authority chief executive asked:

> 'Our question is – is it useful to say, "Here's £x million, now get on with it"? It is much better to have joint discussion on services and priorities. We need to do it around services where change is going on, and not just base it on staff groups.'

The purchasers asked for more detailed service descriptions and wanted measurable outcomes indicated for each service. The Trust pointed out some of the practical difficulties in doing this, but nonetheless agreed to undertake this for some services – physiotherapy, health promotion and family planning. At the next meeting, it emerged that the health authority was looking to break the contract down into nine quantified service sections, with detailed descriptions. The Trust objected to this, arguing that they had previously only agreed in principle to prepare specifications for three of their services. Trust staff argued that each service had different budgets and it was difficult to disentangle them, that there were still major gaps in their information base, and that the purchasers were demanding 'fundamental work'. The purchaser director of contracting pointed out that they were 'starting from a baseline of not knowing what goes on in community . . . If we know some of this, it will enhance the case for investing and changing the service'. Purchasers also wanted to check the allocation of Trust resources to GP fundholders as compared with those going to non-fundholders. The purchaser director of contracting stressed that he had 'no idea about the current disposition of nursing services across the city, its volume and range. It's a closed book'. A compromise was reached in which as much detail as was possible would be provided by the Trust, and more work would be scheduled for later in the year.

Subsequent meetings were completely dominated by arguments about funding levels and the likely impact of further cost reductions on services. Specifications, as such, were not explicitly raised as an issue in the final contract negotiation meetings in 1995. Eventually the contract document was signed in March with further work on the specifications yet to be completed.

In interviews during mid-1995, a purchaser consultant in public health observed that the specifications which were selected were not determined by either the purchasing plan or health needs assessment. They were chosen partly for pragmatic reasons, partly because they were discrete and information was available. The work was 'purchaser-sponsored' and was trying to describe services, see what they cost, define the inputs and outputs – but they were only at 'stage one' in that process. He emphasized that: 'For any of the community services, there is an overwhelming drive to justify the money that we're spending on those services.' He accepted that some services which were 'multi-faceted' (for example health visiting, which can deal with a wide range of functions on one visit) were difficult to specify, but some acute hospital services were equally problematic.

The purchaser assistant director of primary care believed that it was very important to reach a 'shared understanding' about what district nurses and health visitors did, and that this required a joint approach with the Trust. However, she felt that it had not yet been done systematically, nor had specifications been embodied in the formal contract. The director of primary care had taken the lead in 'progress chasing' this joint work and believed that a satisfactory statement had emerged. Initial drafts by the Trust were thought to be inadequate, as they were largely job descriptions and about what was currently provided rather than about needs, but the purchaser wanted much more reference to measurable outcomes.

After prolonged discussions, an agreed set of specifications was produced. The insistence on having more explicit specifications, according to the purchaser director of contracting, came from the purchaser's determination to have greater clarity and accountability: 'because we're not very certain about what they do, what they achieve, what the level of services and resources are'.

From the Trust's perspective there were ambivalent feelings about the health authority's approach to specifications. According to the Trust's director of contracting, there was a lot of rhetoric about the influence of the purchasing plan on specifications, but in reality local circumstances (especially organizational restructuring within the health authority and Trust workload pressures) meant that progress had been slow. Interim specifications had resulted from joint discussions with the purchaser but he was disappointed at their 'low level of sophistication . . . We would have liked them to be more sophisticated, more imaginative . . . rather than just describing what the service is now'. He stressed that community services were *not* so easily identifiable as acute hospital services, and that added to the problem: purchasers can 'see' a hospital ward, patients and operations, but they cannot 'see' the work of health promotion or domiciliary nurses. In contrast with health authorities, GP fundholders had a much better understanding and appreciation of community nursing work, and were less concerned about detailed specification.

These points were repeated by the Trust chief executive, who acknowledged that specifications had been done 'from a professional point of view . . . [about] . . . the way the service is provided now, rather than a specification which is about a new approach'. The services which were selected for detailed descriptions were discrete, activity and costs were relatively easy to identify, and they comprised an integrated service. Others, such as the much larger and more organizationally diverse service like district nursing, were more difficult, and so had been deferred.

Summarizing, it can be concluded that in Area 2, compared with Area 1 there was much more explicit debate about the necessity for commonly agreed specifications (especially during contract negotiations), yet in the same way there had been little substantial progress. The purchaser placed considerable emphasis on the role of specifications in justifying the commitment of resources through contracts, whereas the Trust, though accepting the importance of more precision, stressed the practical limitations of obtaining it.

Area 3

As with the other two areas, in 1993 there was a block contract (see p. 11) which was based on previous service levels and funding. According to the Trust's contracts manager, this contained 'very broad brush' attempts at specifications, which were 'fairly meaningless'. Both the Trust director of finance and the director of contracting wanted to move away from block contracts, since they placed an unfair burden on the provider to meet ever-rising demand without additional funding. This Trust had also done extensive work on building up contracts with GP fundholders in their local area, and accepted the need to tailor-make practice-based provision. They were keen to review and refine their current specifications for both the health authority and GP fundholders.

In November 1993, the health authority purchasers announced that they wanted to influence more closely the kinds of services provided by the Trust and to relate it to purchasing plan objectives and targets. In particular, there was a demand to design outcome-related contracts for five services. Trust managers queried this but accepted the need for more joint work and sharing of information. However, the Trust director of contracting also argued that the purchasing plan had not yielded a well-thought-out 'needs assessment' to enable them to devise better specifications and budgets.

Contract negotiation meetings in early 1994 were largely dominated by arguments about the money the purchaser was prepared to offer, and Trust challenges about whether this demonstrated an abandonment of the purchasing plan strategy to shift resources into community services. There was no direct or explicit reference to the question of service specification as such: the principal issue was the amount of activity and its cost in the following year, and to a lesser extent problems of information (discussed further below). In the meantime, there was an agreement to work collaboratively to develop outcome-related contracts later in the year: the purchaser had begun to draw up an outcome-related contract for maternity services but there was no significant concern about other service specifications. A 'quality' specification drafted by the Trust in June 1994 was eventually agreed and attached as an annexe to the main contract.

The next round of purchaser–provider meetings in the autumn opened with health authority representatives informing the Trust that in the next contracting round, they anticipated 'difficult choices' and reduced finance. They wanted to target their investment in particular services and they needed to review specifications. The purchasers asked for more detailed descriptions of various community services; the provider staff thought their list was 'eclectic' and queried their rationale. In reply, the purchaser director of finance observed:

'There is a dilemma. We are pushed to show how we are buying more health gain, but we don't know what we are buying at the moment, so we can't demonstrate health gain. This is just a platform to go to a different type of contract.'

A debate ensued about whether it was appropriate to specify services in terms of client group or base it on staff inputs. Provider managers stressed the organizational complexity of different services, but said that work was underway to draw up specifications for mental health, elderly and family planning services. The purchasers hoped that this could be a joint exercise. At a subsequent internal purchaser meeting, it was acknowledged that, so far, discussions of specifications had not been part of the formal contract negotiation process, but should be.

In the following round of meetings, the purchasers asked that each service's specifications should include quality items in addition to the separate annexe on quality in the overall contract: provider staff accepted this. A related issue caused some tension and disagreement however. The purchasers intended to draw up plans for selective investment in named 'service developments' and had already been having informal talks with Trust professional staff. Trust managers were annoyed about this and insisted that all discussions should involve them because of the implications for costs and contracting. The Trust director of contracting insisted: 'It's for the Trust to decide what it wants to provide.'

Meetings in early 1995 were entirely preoccupied with arguments about the extent of purchaser cash withdrawals and a re-investment programme, and their impact on, and distribution between, different services. There was no explicit discussion of specifications, though there were intense arguments about finance, which were inevitably connected with the content and organization of services.

In interviews after the completion of the 1995 contracting round, the Trust director of contracting confirmed that work was still proceeding with specifications, and that their content was heavily influenced by Trust staff because 'the commission staff don't really know or greatly understand the detail of the services we provide'. The impetus to do more detailed work on specifications came from the Trust's own 'self-interest' – they were faced with rising demand and increased costs, so improved specifications would help resource allocation. However, this manager believed that neither the Trust nor the Commission had approached specifying services in a systematic way. The main reason for this was the urgency of other issues on their agenda. Moreover, there was a view within the Trust's senior management that devising more complex specifications might be unproductive, a 'paper exercise'. Their recent experience had been that the health authority resource allocation and decisions on investment had not been determined through the contracting process. Thus, according to the Trust director of contracting:

'We could spend ages working up a specification and it not mean anything because contracts are about numbers essentially . . . There seems to be no relationship between anything we do quantitatively about services and the contract discussions.'

Significantly, the purchaser director of public health (who had played a key role throughout the contract negotiations) echoed this view. He was unsure how much importance specifications had in the overall contract, but implied that it was negligible. The process of deciding how much money the Trust received was *not* driven by service specifications, he observed. While those specifications which had been developed now formed a useful 'library of statements of obligation', these were disconnected from the budget process. This gap, he argued, was due to the lack of a valid contract 'currency' for community services, and also due to the Department of Health's fixation about annual increases in the efficiency index, which focused on activity, rather than outcomes. The quasi-market system was built on the 'nonsense' of volume-related contracts, and until this changed, specifications would remain of secondary importance. He advocated a move towards outcome-related contracts:

'If you're paying for *patterns of care*, then the service specifications would become much more important . . . and become the currency of the payment.'

The purchaser chief executive was similarly disappointed at the apparent lack of progress in refining specifications. He thought that there had been examples of good work in jointly planning services with the providers, but this 'was not led by a clear strategic overview of what the contracting intentions are around community services'. This sense of frustration extended to a deeper regret about the lack of development in *commissioning*. The chief executive was aware that money and activity figures had dominated contract negotiations, and that broader service objectives had been eclipsed. While criticizing this situation, he believed there were genuine pragmatic reasons to account for it: 'People start from where we are now, in terms of cost, money, activity, and then [this] approach tends to characterize the annual contracting round.'

It is evident that in Area 3 there was a broad consensus about the need for more detailed specifications, there was broad acceptance of those currently available and they did not appear to be especially contentious issues in negotiations. Most significantly, both provider and purchaser senior managers shared the view that specifications had not had very much impact on the content of the contract, although both parties hoped that they might become more influential in a different contracting regime. In general, it can concluded that Area 3 displayed a similar pattern of experience to Area 1 in that specifications were not major issues of dispute and were perceived to have had little effect on the contracting process. In Area 2, by contrast, specifications were one of several issues of contention and arguments about them were deeply embedded in broader disagreements about resources.

Finance and resources

In any contractual relationship, it can be assumed that having identified what it is that the purchaser wishes to buy, and what the provider can supply, the next most crucial issue in the transaction is the terms of exchange, the agreement on payment for products or services of a prescribed quantity and quality. Commissioning in the NHS ultimately must be expressed in expenditure and the commitment or withdrawal of resources to stimulate competitive efficiency and improved performance. Not surprisingly, discussions about money dominated the interactions between health authorities and Trusts in all three case-study areas. Finance, or more broadly resources, were the constant preoccupations of all those engaged in the contract process. There were, of course, some variations in the intensity with which they were debated, which broadly reflected the specific financial position of each district and its historic pattern of NHS resourcing, but which also derived from the organizational configurations of purchasers and providers, and the particular strategy or stance adopted by the parties. To illustrate this, we shall again examine qualitative evidence by area.

Area 1

In 1993, the health authority's purchasing plan had indicated that, owing to per capita funding reductions and an expressed intention to target certain specific objectives to obtain health gain, it needed to withdraw some funding from all providers, and 're-invest' it in a 'health-improvement programme' linked to health needs assessment priorities. At a commissioning meeting with the CHS provider in March 1993, purchasers emphasized that the Trust could not 'bid against a pot of money', but must suggest which services money could be removed from, and where best it could be redirected. The Trust argued that the greatest unmet needs were in disability services, but the purchaser chief executive demanded further details and their financial implications, adding that 'the bottom line for us is price and volume'. Providers agreed to draw up schemes for possible savings and reinvestment, reassured in the expectation that community services would be overall beneficiaries of a strategic shift away from acute hospital-based services.

By the autumn of 1993, some of the problems of implementing the health-improvement strategy were appearing as providers questioned funding with-drawals. According to the purchaser director of performance management, the 'depressing financial scenario' had posed problems in trying to persuade the community Trust that it would gain in contract terms. The expectation of even more reductions in regional allocations exacerbated the difficulties: providers were now insisting that if the health authority wanted to reduce contract prices, then it must identify the services it did not want to buy, and there were adverse political implications to be considered.

At the next commissioning group meeting, the Trust identified a number of services (various therapy services but especially speech therapy, and com-munity nursing work for community care assessments) where rising demand had caused severe pressure. The Trust chief executive stressed how difficult it was to control CHS activity and caseloads. The purchaser chief executive asked for more detailed information to be supplied: 'If you give us the evidence, that will help us in negotiating the contracts.' However, this prompted an argu-ment about the collection and reporting of routine activity information, with the Trust arguing that it was unable to comply with the purchaser's requests because their information system was inadequate, and they needed extra fund-ing for new computer systems.

Subsequent contract negotiation meetings concluded in mutually accept-able decisions about finance and activity. According to the Trust chief execu-tive, the eventual contract did yield additional income, and there was also extra income from GP fundholders, so there was some financial security. For the health authority purchasers, one important concern was to get providers to accept the principle that there was now a 'volume-sensitive' contract, and that any variation (in activity) had to be agreed by both parties, and the volume must be 'managed' by the Trust within the contract price. Again the providers noted that there were technical problems in measuring activity and in switching between 'underperforming' and 'overperforming' services, but the point was acceded.

At one of the mid-year commissioning group meetings, Trust managers listed a number of services where they had experienced increased demand and a growing inability to deal with the workload. Waiting lists were getting longer, and the Trust had begun to devise internal professional protocols to prioritize needs, especially in community paediatric nursing and chiropody.

Purchasers responded by asking for documentation and more detailed evidence; they also asked whether possible staff restrictive practices had been overcome and if skill-mix solutions were feasible. It was pointed out that the Trust had benefited financially from the recent health-improvement programme and the purchasers still had doubts about the accuracy of the Trust's information on activity.

By the end of 1994, arguments about funding became more pronounced, worsened by the fact that the purchasing plan required a substantial deduction of money from all local providers. At a tense and unusually conflictual commissioning meeting in December, the provider director of contracting criticized this policy and asked purchasers which services they expected them to 'disinvest' from. Purchasers described the policy as not so much a withdrawal, more a 're-direction' of resources. Once more the Trust identified several services which needed additional funding due to increased demand, and complained angrily about current cash-flow problems owing to delays in receiving payments from the health authority.

Finance and resources were clearly the most pressing concern internally for the purchaser too. A senior management team meeting in January 1995 discussed various ways of obtaining (as the chief executive put it) the most 'bangs for bucks' – maximizing activity and reaching the Department of Health efficiency index target. They established their basic position for negotiating with providers; each provider would be offered a 2.7 per cent increase in finance over the existing contract value, in return for a 4 per cent increase in activity. If the Trusts disagreed, then the health authority would 're-base' (that is, change the value) of the contracts.

At a negotiation meeting in January 1995, despite reservations about the validity of activity information and alternative ways of reaching the efficiency target, the Trust agreed to accept an offer based on a 2.7 per cent increase in funding for a 3 per cent overall increase in activity, and an assurance from the purchaser that they would receive more money, but targeted on specific services. The outline contract was agreed and signed at a meeting a few weeks later with very little further discussion.

It later emerged that this initial agreement was withdrawn by the Trust because the health authority had awarded additional funding to acute hospital providers and another mixed hospital-and-community service provider, to help reduce their waiting lists. The Trust argued that these decisions had been taken outside of contract negotiations, and should have formed part of the formal discussion of resources; they threatened to go to arbitration. Eventually the health authority agreed to release extra funding to the Trust to offset some of their service pressures, but Trust managers still felt aggrieved about the incident, and suggested that it revealed the purchasers had 'succumbed' to acute hospitals' demands by giving them preferential allocations. The issue was perceived as fundamental to the Trust's confidence in the purchasers' integrity, and it was especially important given the Trust's increasing difficulty in meeting rising demand.

Senior purchasing managers' overriding concern was ensuring that there was sufficient money overall to pay for *all* current contracts – 'affordability' was the biggest problem. The main sticking point in negotiations, according to the director of contracting, was that 'the community unit [*sic*] would like us to fund more than we can afford. And they've got a point: there *are* pressures in the community'. There was some frustration that while the purchaser wanted to develop CHS, there were insufficient resources. Other informants acknowledged that they had difficulty in demonstrating that they had been 'even-handed' with different providers, and one observed that the resolution of the financial dispute was the 'usual' NHS 'fudge and mudge'.

Thus, for Area 1 financial and resource issues had been at the core of their discussions. While the first round of contracting produced a mutually acceptable agreement, the second round appeared to yield a satisfactory bargain which was then partially confounded by decisions taken outside of the contracting arena. For the providers, as we shall note later, this soured what they had believed previously to be a cooperative relationship.

Area 2

Area 2 had a number of distinctive features, because there had been a merger of three former districts into one DHA, the amalgamation of several community units to form one large CHS Trust, and there was current controversy over possible 'rationalization' of several large acute hospitals. Compared to the other two case-study areas, the purchasing power of Area 2 was much larger, but owing to per capita funding reductions, they had the most difficult financial position. The 1993 purchasing plan anticipated zero growth in real terms funding and wanted to shift the balance of resources away from secondary to primary and community sectors.

During contract negotiations in early 1993, the purchaser sought changes in the value of the current CHS block contract so that the Trust increased activity by 1.5 per cent and made additional 1 per cent internal cost savings. The Trust opposed this, stressing the growth in demand for their services, and warning that they would have to make real service reductions as well as defer developments. The purchasers were anxious about the service implications, but accepted a package of proposals made by the Trust. The Trust's view was that the health authority had not fulfilled their strategy of shifting resources into community services, and consequently, in the words of the director of contracting, 'the service is being squeezed,' with community nursing taking the brunt of reductions.

In the summer of 1993, the purchaser debated its next purchasing plan and considered how they might protect CHS from the effect of further funding reductions and so prevent more service reductions. Some argued that hospitals and the community trust should be treated similarly, whereas others favoured 'ring-fencing' CHS. A decision was taken to seek higher cost savings targets from above-average-cost acute specialties. Following this, disquiet among health authority members about the impact on acute hospitals led to the abandonment of the attempt to protect CHS funding. Purchaser managers were dismayed at this decision and noted that it would create severe problems in the next contract negotiations and in prioritizing bids from providers for service developments.

It also contradicted the position purchasers outlined to the Trust in their regular 'liaison group' meetings in the summer of 1993. Purchaser representatives had already assured the Trust that CHS were given priority, though all providers were being asked to find extra resources from internal efficiency savings. Trust managers emphasized that savings could only be obtained through staff losses, and this was counterproductive, especially since they were already 'overstretched'.

Financial pressures were the major item of discussion in subsequent meetings. The Trust reported that they had asked all their heads of service to identify schemes for more savings without affecting clinical services, but this was extremely difficult. The purchaser director of contracting observed:

'We live in a world where we want to provide services effectively but resources are constrained. If you think the measures will have a perceptible impact on services, you should discuss them: it's a *shared* concern.'

The Trust gave detailed examples of the effects of budget reductions on various elements of their work, like increased waiting lists and the inevitable slowing down of hospital discharges.

At the next contract negotiation meeting, the purchaser told the Trust that they had to achieve a 2 per cent efficiency gain and other cost savings, and that they wanted a block contract with 'floors and ceilings'. Once again the Trust chief executive stressed the probable effect of reductions on the continuity of care and argued that the purchasing plan appeared to ignore other health needs which CHS should be meeting. A very similar discussion occurred at the next liaison group meeting. The Trust listed all their internal efficiency measures, and also tabled a list of current pressures leading to overspending. Responding to purchaser requests to achieve an efficiency target of 2 per cent, the Trust managers argued that first, owing to inadequate information systems, activity and thus efficiency could not be measured accurately, and second, if cuts were to be made, it would affect work for GPs, community care and hospital discharge rates. The purchaser representatives insisted that the Trust must prepare plans to cope with rising demand and fund pressures internally.

Further meetings constantly revisited these issues, with little sign of movement by either side, although purchasers stressed that they needed to have a detailed understanding of possible service reductions, so that they could 'stand together, rather than blame each other'. Trust managers reported that they were trying to protect community nursing and frontline services, but were taking money out of all other budgets, including health visiting. Pressed to spell out the scale of these reductions, Trust representatives were reluctant to describe exactly how they were to be implemented, to the annoyance of purchaser staff.

By February 1994, it was apparent that there was a large shortfall in health authority funding and the Trust's requirements. This had been exacerbated by the additional costs of Trust amalgamation with other CHS units and historic problems of underfunding. The Trust informed the purchaser that they would be unable to meet their activity target, and that pressures on the service could only be met through cuts elsewhere in their budget. The purchasers insisted that if there were service reductions, these would have to be agreed with them. The purchaser director of contracting stated that he could not recommend that the health authority sign the proposed contract with the Trust's planned cuts, so he anticipated going to arbitration.

There appeared to be stalemate, and in the words of one informant, 'It will be a miracle if we get any contract at all'. Eventually there was arbitration by the regional health authority. The deadlock was broken by providing some additional special finance for the Trust, a compromise about activity targets which deferred agreement about the 'baseline', and an 'understanding' about possible service reductions. To an observer, the atmosphere among both purchaser and Trust managers, throughout these negotiations, was fraught, stressed and tense.

Largely as a result of this experience, a new purchaser–provider group was established (in the summer of 1994) to debate strategy as well as to deal with contract negotiations. Almost the first item for discussion was the financial situation 1994–5. The Trust chief executive said that there was serious underfunding and financial problems. Purchasers asked for a 'complete picture, holding nothing back' but reminded the providers that the health authority itself had major funding problems and was expecting all Trusts to lower their contract prices. The Trust reported that they had made service reductions of about £1 million and had embarked on other 'rationalizations'. Purchasers asked for an assessment of the effects, service by service, but Trust representatives replied that their information system prevented them from doing this. Purchasers interpreted this as being uncooperative and obstinate. Seeking an accommodation, the purchaser director of public health noted:

> 'Even if you're having problems in measuring activity, we need at least to *share* information on inputs . . . We have to describe together what has happened to community services, so that we can work out a way to get more money. We need to think laterally and imaginatively. At least let's share it.'

Similarly, the purchaser director of contracting said:

> 'We are sympathetic, but it comes across as though you are not wanting to share this information with us. What can we do? We can only assume that in the absence of evidence, the cuts have not had much impact – and this must affect our contract position.'

Trust staff argued that they were not being difficult or uncooperative, but there were technical and staffing problems in obtaining and collating the necessary information. It was agreed to do more work to identify the impact of cost savings, and the purchaser chief executive again emphasized, 'You expect us to trust you about the alleged underfunding, but you need to *show* us'.

Three subsequent meetings of this group were dominated by discussion of financial issues. The Trust outlined the progress it was making with service reductions and described the 'inherited pressures' which were causing overspending again. Purchasers indicated that their purchasing plan was based on securing more provider-generated savings and wanted the Trust to share more information with them about their current business position and strategic plans. The purchaser director of contracting noted that he could not see much 'common ground' in their search to generate the £1 million needed for developments. At the December meeting, the purchasers told the Trust that they had to increase activity levels by 3 per cent, but the expected regional financial allocation was 'bad news' – further savings of £3 million had to be achieved. This was a change from their purchasing plan and previous expectations. There were also separate 'purchaser pressures' on the Trust budget of £2 million, and Trust service development plans for £2 million. Not surprisingly, the Trust managers reacted with shock at this announcement, and purchasers tried to persuade them of the need to agree another radical cost savings programme.

By January 1995, the situation had changed significantly, as the regional allocation was better than anticipated, giving some money for growth which could be used to offset pressures and developments. The purchasers' position was that they now would not reduce the value of the contract, but they did want to 'validate' the Trust's claims about cost pressures, and to check that they had maximized their efficiency savings. The Trust confirmed that they would be able to meet the activity target, though they were still concerned about underfunding, and stressed the difficulties they were having in meeting demand; they also pointed out that they would not be able to fulfil some of the *Patient's Charter* and other quality aspects of the contract. The provider chief executive cautioned that, 'we're accepting a considerable burden of coping with internal pressures, and I hope that's understood'. The purchaser director of finance replied: '*All* providers . . . have to cope, but there's not a lot of room for manoeuvre'.

During the next three negotiation meetings, the purchasers offered some extra finance but demanded a detailed schedule of Trust cost pressures and the measures they were taking to deal with them. This demand was resisted by the Trust, but purchasers insisted that the Trust should justify their claims for resources, and urged them to do more work to find additional efficiency savings. Trust representatives argued that efficiency measures actually had adverse effects on services and would lead to the loss of staff. At points during several of these meetings, the purchasers withdrew temporarily for private talks, and then offered other ways of dealing with what had become an impasse. The deadline for signing contracts was approaching, but no agreement seemed likely. The purchasers affirmed that there was no more money available, so the Trust had to find ways of resolving its financial problems internally. The purchaser director of contracting observed that 'There is a gap in understanding between us, and a gap in substance'.

By mid-February 1995, the Trust had drawn up another list of further cost-saving measures, but it still fell short of their total budget requirements. The purchasers noted that there was still a major gap between the parties, and no solution was in sight. They wanted explicit assurances about what the extra funding they had offered would buy in the next year, they wanted compliance with the quality standards, and no service reductions. Another extra amount of cash was offered for one year only, to assist the Trust with its special difficulties.

The Trust managers replied that they could not guarantee there would be no service reductions, and while recognizing the extra cash offer, stated that it was still insufficient to enable them to deliver the contract. After more protracted debate and argument, the Trust chief executive announced that the board had authorized him to sign the contract for activity and finance, but to add a caveat about necessary service reductions, which would be made public. A final decision was postponed to later meetings of the negotiation group.

At those meetings, there were lengthy and detailed discussions of alternative options proposed by the Trust, and their likely financial effect; both parties appeared to be looking for a compromise. The purchasers' view was that there had been some progress, the Trust had shifted its position, but the purchasers were still dissatisfied that insufficient money had been found internally, and they objected to planned service reductions. The Trust chief executive reminded them that community nursing had previously borne the brunt of cuts and could not sustain rising demand and increased throughput from acute hospitals. At the end of February, a compromise agreement was provisionally reached, in which increases in activity to conform with the efficiency gain requirement were accepted, some service 'rationalizations' and reductions were acknowledged, and a joint purchaser–provider project group was to be set up to achieve a balanced budget throughout the rest of the financial year.

Reviewing this second round of negotiations, the Trust director of finance thought that the agreement was not to any of the parties' satisfaction, therefore it probably represented a fair result. The contract had placed severe constraints on Trust finances, and they were anticipating very difficult internal decisions coping with further cost savings. The director of contracting said that their principal objectives had been to minimize the reduction in their contract income, and minimize increases in activity. It had been a 'battle' – negotiations had been 'very difficult', 'very entrenched' – but overall they believed that they had secured those objectives. The Trust chief executive felt that the major sticking points were entirely financial, and reflected the purchaser's *adversarial* determination to focus on cost and price without appreciating the Trust's arguments about service implications. The concentration on activity and money obscured a better understanding of services and had led to feelings of distrust on both sides.

From the purchasers' perspective, some informants thought that although the health authority had secured its objective of getting more activity for the same, or less resources, the contract did not develop and improve community services. They accepted that they had sometimes adopted assertive or even confrontational stances in negotiations, and that this had antagonized the Trust and had been unproductive. One respondent regretted that they had not got a contract which genuinely maintained previous service levels, and criticized the 'fudging' of decisions about cost improvement measures by the Trust; there was also a concern that the Trust had withheld information thereby weakening their credibility.

A key figure in the negotiations claimed that the sticking points in negotiations were not essentially 'financial' but were rather about *resources*. For this purchaser:

'It's about the services provided in relation to the resources, because the negotiation is about both sides of the equation.'

He emphasized that their style of negotiations was the same for all of the provider Trusts (including large acute hospitals) they contracted with, but acknowledged that he had expected the CHS contract to be one of the most difficult. He also recognized that at important phases, purchasers had been 'adversarial' and 'tough-minded': there had been a 'logjam' and lack of progress which eventually had to be overcome.

Thus it can be seen that in Area 2, finance and resources were overwhelmingly important. Although purchaser–provider relationships were not personally antagonistic, there were fundamental divisions (and some mutual suspicion and mistrust) between the Trust and the health authority about the contract, temporarily 'resolved' by an unsatisfactory compromise for both parties.

Area 3

The purchaser in Area 3 had a high profile in commissioning, and its purchasing plan strategy had signalled a shift in resources away from acute hospitals into primary and community services. It had a three-year rolling block contract with the CHS Trust, but wanted to move towards more sophisticated contracts. At purchaser–provider meetings in November 1993, the purchasers announced that they expected there to be significant losses of income for the community contract in the next year, but the health authority expected to buy the same 'basket of goods' as in the previous year. The Trust vigorously challenged these resource assumptions and financial calculations.

At meetings in February 1994, the purchasers gave more details of their demands: they had received an increased allocation of almost 3 per cent, but proposed only a 2.2 per cent increase to the Trust, with a requirement for increased activity. This was keenly disputed by the Trust representatives, who argued that the purchaser was not fulfilling its purchasing plan commitment, that purchasers would spend proportionately more on the local acute hospital Trust and that the CHS Trust would not deliver more activity for less funding. Virtually identical arguments were voiced at the next meeting, with providers arguing that the purchaser should pass on the full financial allocation. If they did not, it would indicate that they had *not* given priority to CHS as promised in the purchasing plan.

Further meetings failed to resolve the disagreement, but private talks between purchaser and provider chief executives were held in order to avoid having to go to arbitration, and a compromise offer was made. Trust managers pragmatically accepted the additional cash offer but felt aggrieved. They believed that the purchaser had reneged on earlier undertakings to enhance and support community services, in the face of demands from the acute hospital Trust. As one provider informant put it: 'The purchasing plan has no credibility, and now I don't believe anything the purchaser tells me . . . We will do what the letter of the contract says, and no more.' In practice, the Trust was able to stabilize its finances by gaining extra GP fundholder income and internal efficiency measures, but the widely held view was that the purchasers had failed to honour their published commitment to community services.

In the autumn of 1994, the purchasers informed the Trust that their opening position for negotiations was that they would not buy any more activity, but would withdraw cash from the contract and re-invest it in selected service developments. The purchaser director of finance warned the Trust that 'There will be difficult choices and decisions to be made'. Replying to a Trust manager's question about abandoning the policy of switching resources into CHS, the director of finance denied this, assuring them it was really an attempt to get 'measured investments'. This policy of disinvestment and re-investment caused more heated exchanges in the next meeting: provider representatives complained about chronic underfunding and reported that there was staff anxiety about future cuts, and anger about the purchasers' obvious protection of the acute hospital Trust. Another meeting became acrimonious as provider managers disputed the purchasers' logic of asking Trust professional staff to prepare bids for service developments when the purchaser was at the same time making a 2.75 per cent cash withdrawal.

In meetings in January 1995, both sides appeared conciliatory but the major obstacle was the purchasers' demand to inspect and approve the Trust's internal schemes for generating efficiency and cost savings. As a purchaser representative expressed it: 'You have to satisfy us that it's genuine efficiency – tell us now that there is cash on the table . . . If you can't fund the service developments with [your efficiency savings] money, then we must make painful choices.'

Trust managers suggested possible cost-saving schemes, but also indicated their negative effects on patients, staff and workloads. With great reluctance, and after much pressure by the purchaser, they agreed to submit a list of potential internal savings. The purchasers were determined to ensure that the Trust had exhausted all internal sources in their search for revenue, and were reluctant to disclose in which types of service the health authority would prefer to see limited 're-investment'. One of the key figures in the purchaser team put it bluntly: 'You produce a plan to show how you can fund the service priorities you have, and then show the pain [from cash withdrawals in the contract] – then we can negotiate.'

A few weeks later, the health authority's financial situation had improved because of a more generous regional allocation than was expected. At negotiation meetings, however, the Trust again described the severity of their budget problems and the purchasers criticized their apparent intransigence. The leading negotiator for the purchaser insisted that the Trust should inform them about the choices made inside the provider (about how they would manage expenditure reductions) saying: 'We want to drive you hard, to get as great value-for-money . . . We want an open-book approach.' Provider representatives argued that service cuts and more efficiency measures would demoralize their professional staff, and stressed that they could not achieve a 2.75 per cent reduction. A stalemate had been reached and negotiations were temporarily suspended.

In mid-February, as the deadline for contract signing approached, it emerged that (as in the previous year) a compromise settlement was fixed by purchaser and provider chief executives outside of the formal negotiating teams. The health authority increased the cash value of its offer, and the Trust accepted a contract for activity and finance. Further meetings took place through March to finalize plans for funding service developments in line with purchaser priorities.

In later interviews, most purchasers expressed the view that they had achieved their objectives. However, a senior manager acknowledged that both purchaser and provider had become antagonistic and some of the negotiations had become 'truly adversarial'. Financial problems had predominated to the detriment of strategic debate about services.

In the provider, by May 1995 feelings were still negative: several informants thought that the final outcome was reasonably favourable for the Trust, but the contract negotiation process had created mistrust and bitterness. They criticized apparent changes and inconsistencies in the purchasers' position, and felt that their behaviour was in marked contrast to that of other purchasers they had dealt with, whom they regarded as more honest and open. One informant observed that the Trust now felt vulnerable because their main purchaser had often behaved in a 'bizarre' way during negotiations. While the final agreement on money was broadly satisfactory to the Trust, it was perceived as arbitrary rather than rational, and the experience had damaged working relationships between the Trust and the purchaser.

Conclusions

This chapter has presented case-study findings about the two most fundamental aspects of the contracting process: defining the content of the services being commissioned and setting the financial terms on which services are purchased. It has been shown that regarding specifications, in general there were conscious attempts to develop and refine the description of services, but that few if any of the parties believed that such specifications were decisively important in their contractual relationship.

In Area 1, the health authority began by trying to improve the specifications, and although this did not produce conflict with the provider, there was little progress; by mid-1995, there was an accommodation with the provider simply to do further work. In Area 2, the purchaser similarly declared that it wanted much more detailed specifications; in contrast to Area 1, this did provoke provider objections, mainly about the level of detail demanded by the health authority. Specifications thus emerged as a focus for continuing disagreement. For the Trust, the purchasers' insistence on prescriptive specifications indicated their lack of understanding of the nature of CHS. For the purchaser, there was an assumption that the Trust was constantly withholding information, and so specifications were the principal method for ensuring contract compliance. Purchasers thought that the task of drawing up CHS specifications were, theoretically at least, no different from those for acute hospital services, but the providers argued that community services were special and problematic. Both parties believed that the specifications which finally did emerge were not the outcome of a systematic needs assessment or outcome-oriented process.

In Area 3, the purchasers wanted outcome-related contracts, and the Trust indicated its willingness to assist in their design, seeing it as a way of managing risk and avoiding excess demand. While in 1993–4, specifications did not appear as a significant issue, they became contentious in the 1994–5 contracting round. However, neither the purchaser nor the provider believed that specifications had played an important role in shaping the final contract; this was effectively determined by finance.

Indeed, arguments over finance and resources dominated contract negotiations in each area. In Area 1, the recurring issue was whether the Trust's claims about increased and unresourced workload could be adequately documented. In 1994–5, the key issue was how to reconcile the Trust's demands for additional funding with the health authority's strategy of disinvesting in some services and re-investing in other priorities. What seemed like a mutually-acceptable and successful negotiation was then disrupted by a dispute over money after the outline contract had been signed. This was perceived by the providers as having undermined an otherwise cooperative relationship.

In Area 2, financial difficulties were overwhelmingly dominant in both contracting rounds. At each stage of negotiations there were lengthy arguments about the scale and nature of service reductions necessary to cope with the purchasers' contract offer, and accusations by the Trust that the health authority had abandoned its purchasing plan commitments to improve CHS provision. The purchasers' earnest intention to protect CHS could not be sustained. They experienced constant frustration trying to persuade the Trust to demonstrate precisely how they would manage reduced funding. Their perception was that the Trust was unwilling to 'share' information, and this then hampered the purchasers' efforts to justify the commitment of extra resources.

In Area 3 finance was also the most significant issue: in both contracting rounds, the Trust argued that the purchaser had failed to implement its stated policy of moving resources into community services. Despite reaching satisfactory compromises about funding after initial stalemates in *both* contracting rounds, there was intense resentment among Trust managers that no substantial shift in resources had occurred. There was also deep suspicion among providers about the purchasers forcing the Trust to open its accounts (to show all the internal cost-saving measures it was taking) before it was permitted to receive investment money for some service developments. Even purchaser informants acknowledged that financial issues had obscured strategic policy objectives and had generated unnecessary conflict.

In many ways these experiences are in line with findings from other studies of the contracting process. The National Audit Office's (1995) study found that hospitals and health authorities were still 'mainly concerned with achieving their own distinct objectives rather than coming to a jointly beneficial agreement' (1995: 19) and that acute services contract negotiations tended to focus on changes in the total *price* of the contract and total patient activity. Many of the issues described above are also reported as being common in most other types of NHS contracting (Appleby 1994): the preoccupation with the efficiency index, the very slow development away from block contracts, problems in obtaining reliable information to measure performance and difficulties in devising contract currencies linked to outcomes.

Clearly, what they also show among purchasers is an oscillation in styles, moving between *adversarial* and *collaborative* modes of negotiation at different times and over different issues. Official guidance recommends 'an atmosphere of creative tension rather than a cosy relationship which inhibits change' (National Audit Office 1995: 19) and in all three case-study areas, the health authorities can be seen to have adopted assertive or directive styles towards their main CHS providers. At the same time, there were frequent references to the necessity and merits of 'joint' working, 'shared understandings' and cooperative strategies, coinciding with other official guidance to promote local health alliances and 'mature' long-term relationships (NHS Management Executive 1990; Key *et al.* 1994; Hancock 1995).

What is also evident, however, is that owing to the inherent features of community health services – their local boundedness, pattern of delivery and high level of discretionary content – mainstream CHS provision tended to come from a local near-monopoly supplier and purchasers were both reluctant and unable to consider radical changes or cancellation of contracts. Problems in measuring activity and in evaluating effectiveness constrained most purchasers to working with block contracts (with some ceilings and floors) but this did not prevent them from attempting to secure more control over specifications and from trying to impose their own commissioning priorities on Trust service developments and schemes for cost reductions.

In making those attempts, however, there were episodes when their motives and actions were seen as dogmatic or threatening by providers, and this had the effect of weakening the assumed affinities and mutuality which most CHS Trusts believed they shared with the purchasers, and which they presumed carried weight in the purchasing plan and contracting process.

The importance of 'relational markets' discussed in Chapter 1, was recognised by all parties, and there seemed to be a genuine desire to construct a 'partnership' model of contracting, but the frequently adversarial character of many of the contract negotiations tended to erode the essential component of trust. As Propper (1993) and Propper *et al.* (1994) suggested, where there is no competitive market, and/or there are doubts about compliance with quality requirements, purchasers can either rely on trust or they can try to stipulate specifications in great detail. Ferlie (1994) found that in the acute sector, such trust had not yet evolved: the relationship between purchasers and providers was 'negotiative rather than fully cooperative' (1994: 221).

In this case study, purchasers veered between hard and soft approaches to contracting. Central government instructions to promote contestability, accountability and value for money ultimately came to dominate their commissioning and contracting approach. The effect was often to corrode rather than nurture common values and commitments, to create an atmosphere of mistrust and to exacerbate inherent problems of uncertainty in the contract process.

7

Monitoring contracts:
negotiating performance
and quality

The development of the NHS internal market and contracts required a complex system of monitoring, to ensure that the services delivered by providers matched those demanded by purchasers. While the emphasis on monitoring was not new, it took a different form and became institutionalized in the contracting process. Throughout the 1980s, the NHS had experienced the application of a wide range of surveillance instruments, and new methods of inspection and evaluation (Flynn 1992a). Quasi-markets – the putative move away from bureaucratic hierarchy to competitive contracts – intensified central government's insistence on further controls on accountability and value for money (Harrison 1993).

In the initial official guidance on contracts, adequate monitoring arrangements were regarded as vital, as contracts could only be effective if their performance could be assessed. It was also noted that such monitoring might take time to develop (because of problems in measuring quality) and that systems should not become unwieldy and impractical. Ultimately, monitoring could be used by purchasers in improving contract specifications and in identifying where alternative or additional providers might be necessary (Department of Health 1989c). Further guidance stressed that the establishment of quality standards was a 'critical issue' in the contracting process and the onus was upon providers to demonstrate precisely how they were meeting the purchasers' requirements. Information was necessary 'to verify that the contract is being met in quantity and quality terms' (NHS Management Executive 1990b: 6, 19). It was recognized that while appropriate measures of quality were still evolving, quantifiable measures were preferred: 'there is little point in specifying standards of performance for contracts unless their achievement can be monitored' (1990: 30). Although in general it was accepted that penalties that punish providers for non-performance were 'inappropriate', health authorities were urged to ensure that there were *remedies* and *disincentives* for non-performance.

These views conform with conventional economic theories of contracting, where information 'asymmetry' is regarded as a major threat to efficient competition. However, the 'lack of observability' in the production of health and social care poses special difficulties in regulating quality, where those delivering the service may have a much better knowledge of it than purchasers (Propper 1993; Robinson 1994). Inevitably, there are problems in setting standards and practical difficulties in discovering whether these are attained. During the early phase of the market reforms, information technology and computer systems were said to be absent or poor, assessing patient outcomes was problematic and entailed long time periods; record keeping systems were poor and audit procedures were professionally controlled rather than oriented to purchasers (Kerrison 1993). Nevertheless, the monitoring of quality became a principal concern in the Government's policy on market regulation and a burgeoning growth industry for commentators and advisers (Øvretveit 1992, 1995; Gaster 1995).

As we argued in Chapter 1, health authorities encounter severe difficulties in measuring activity, costs and quality in CHS. Nevertheless, in our case-study areas (see Appendix), continuous efforts were made to overcome these difficulties, and both purchasers and providers regarded problems of contract monitoring as important indications of their broader relationship. To illustrate some of these problems, and attempts to resolve them, we shall again consider qualitative evidence drawn from analysis of documents, observational fieldwork and interviews over two contracting rounds in the three areas.

Area 1

The 1994–5 purchasing plan for this area emphasized the importance of developing a 'quality strategy' with all providers, stressing that standards would be mutually agreed. Such standards were to be 'challenging but realistic' and derived from the purchaser's priorities. Of the six examples which were given, three referred to acute hospital issues (for example, reduced waiting times for inpatient treatment) while three referred to 'non-acute' provision (provision of vaccinations, improvement in learning disability services and improved access for people with sensory impairment). Most of the discussion of quality was based on aspects of the national *Patient's Charter* objectives.

The plan emphasized that the purchaser intended to focus on quality outcomes rather than the structures and processes which providers used. Monitoring was expected to be 'meaningful without being over-bureaucratic', achieved through measurable standards which were required in quarterly reports from providers. In order to underline the importance of quality and *Patient's Charter* targets, a 'performance bond' was introduced (the value related to the total contract price). If annual reports were unsatisfactory, money would be withheld for inadequate or non-performance.

In the provider Trust, their business plan stated unequivocally their commitment to improving the quality of provision, and endorsed principles of quality assurance for the whole organization. Quality was expected to be built into all service plans, it was a responsibility for all staff, each profession was expected to define their clinical standards and there was to be an internal procedure for monitoring and reviewing service quality. The overriding importance of national *Patient's Charter* standards was noted (and set out in detail in terms of specific objectives or 'key result areas') but the business plan also added that quality was about 'specifying what is realistic for the Unit'.

This, then, was the broad framework for the evaluation and monitoring of quality. How was it dealt with through the contracting process ? Throughout 1993, when the provider unit was a 'shadow' Trust, the chief executive was concerned about the inadequacy of their information system and their inability to measure activity, costs and workload precisely for district nursing and health visiting. This was regarded as a serious issue and was discussed at regular purchaser–provider meetings. The purchasers had indicated that they wanted to move towards outcome-related contracts, but these required much more sophisticated information than was available. The provider director of contracting accepted the principle of devising outcome-oriented contracts but warned that it was very hard to identify outcomes in CHS because their effects were often long-term and difficult to measure.

In general, quality monitoring was regarded as very slow to develop, and was done informally: 'the purchasers are as confused as we are about how best to measure outcomes'. The provider staff had proposed certain professional service standards to the purchaser and they wanted collaborative work to develop them. A purchaser consultant in public health acknowledged that information was a problem for them, especially about the content and outcomes of health visiting. Quality issues were increasingly important to the purchasers, but in CHS they were restricted mainly to aspects like waiting times for appointments or domiciliary visits and accessibility of clinics. The purchaser director of performance management observed that most of their quality targets were *Patient's Charter* objectives, but this was problematic in CHS because CHS did not fit the 'hard' *Patient's Charter* standards, and thus had to rely on 'softer' indicators. Contract monitoring was principally about analysing variations in planned activity and costs, done through quarterly assessments and meetings. The original estimates of workload built into the block contract (see p. 11) appeared to be inaccurate as well as out of date, so this was causing concern.

The purchaser director of contracting also recognized that there were problems in obtaining reliable and meaningful information, and this was attributed to historical underfunding of CHS – community units had been the 'poor relation' so lacked the administrative infrastructure as well as the investment in computer hardware and software. It was seen as vital not only to get accurate information about activity and costs, but also about effectiveness. This respondent did not regard this as an adversarial position but saw it rather as a collaborative and developmental approach. He favoured a partnership style of contracting: he wanted the provider to describe their business but link it to meaningful measures, and ask, 'if they had not got the information, then how could they develop it?' He stressed: 'We try to work on a "discussion" model rather than a "You will do" model – that's no way of doing contracts.'

This stance was not always reflected in discussions at purchaser–provider meetings, however. At one of their regular meetings, there was a disagreement about the purchaser's demands for activity monitoring. The Trust chief executive insisted that this was a long-standing issue: they could not send the information because they had inadequate resources to collate and analyse the data required. They had not received any funding from the purchaser to assist the routine collection and processing of activity information. The purchaser chief executive replied that they *must* send them the information, and noted that this argument was 'souring our relationship'. A decision was reached to investigate what practical improvements could be made to supply some partial information. Two months later (in November 1993) at another 'contract review' meeting, information and monitoring were again issues of dispute. Purchaser representatives said that they knew the Trust had some problems with information but pressed them for improvements. The Trust managers countered that they had staffing problems as well as insufficient investment in information technology. The purchasers reminded them that they had been talking about these issues for two years and they should have been resolved. They wanted to move to outcome-oriented contracts, so information was vital: the Trust would have to consider other ways of improving their data collection.

By spring 1994, these difficulties were still causing concern. A purchaser–provider contract monitoring meeting debated continuing problems in obtaining information, and they agreed to cooperate to sort out the information system. The importance of this was also noted in a service commissioning meeting, where purchasers warned that unless there were accurate and agreed figures about the activity baseline, they would be 'on quicksand'.

The final signing of the annual contract left the resolution of activity figures for further joint discussion, and there was a separate 'quality' schedule attached as an annexe to the main contract. In interviews in mid-1994, the purchaser DoC maintained that they wanted to develop outcome-based contracts with better quality indicators built in, but this must be done collaboratively with the provider. He did not believe that CHS were intrinsically more difficult to devise outcome measures for, but progress had been slow owing to the inadequate investment in information collection and computer facilities. He wanted future contracts to break the CHS down into components and say what interventions were expected to achieve, to link activity with outcomes and evaluate the effectiveness of their investment. However, this was constrained by information problems. One other related feature of the contract was also designed to improve providers' performance: the purchaser intended to introduce a 'performance bond'. If information was not supplied as required within a specified time period, or if there was a high level of patient complaints, or if the *Patient's Charter* standards were not met, then the purchaser would withhold money (one example was £50 000 on a £16 million contract). This was intended to get providers to build quality into all elements of their operation: 'It's putting the principle in there that quality actually means something, and there's money attached to it.'

The three-year rolling block contract in operation from 1994 contained a statement of quality standards as a separate annexe, detailing 54 minimum national and local standards; 40 of these were intended to apply to *all* providers. The others were particularly for acute hospital and mental health providers. None was *specifically* identified as applying to community health services as such. The contract also outlined the mechanism for monitoring: 'technical' aspects of monitoring were to be dealt with separately at routine meetings to review current performance, while strategic issues were to be discussed at more formal quarterly meetings of a purchaser–provider 'service commissioning forum'.

Significantly, the provider contract negotiations with GP fundholders had resulted in agreement to use the main health authority's quality specifications, amended as necessary for particular practices. The relevant sections of the community nursing quality schedule referred to the Trust ensuring that its staff were adequately trained and qualified, appropriate managerial support was available for staff, every client received an assessment of needs and a seamless service, staff participated in community care planning and care assessments and that clients' cultural needs were considered. References were made to minimum waiting times, appointments for visits to patients, staff adherence to professional codes and standards, and methods for clinical audit. Service-specific issues were listed separately. District nursing, for example, aimed to 'provide nursing support to clients and carers in order that they remain in their own homes and retain independence'. Hours of cover were detailed, together with referral procedures and minimum response times prioritized in terms of urgency. The schedules for health visiting and therapy services had a similar format, and described their aims and objectives as well as operational aspects of service delivery. Procedures for dealing with monitoring, non-performance, variations and arbitration or termination of the contract were also indicated.

Many of these quality considerations were highly generalized and referred to structures and processes, rather than outcomes. However, one contract with the health authority did specifically mention outcomes. The learning disabilities service objectives included: reducing the incidence of challenging behaviour; reducing stress among the carers and families of clients with learning disabilities; increasing self-help skills; and enhancing the quality of life of clients in residential care. The contract noted that targets for these outcomes would be developed and that these would then form a baseline for subsequent monitoring of quality.

This was the formal and procedural aspect of contract monitoring. But how was it implemented in practice? It was evident that purchasers and providers did not conceptualize issues of quality and monitoring as being distinct from any other element in the contracting process. They were inextricably bound up with concerns over information about activity and resources. Thus, for example, in the late summer of 1994, the provider chief executive noted that the health authority seemed to be wanting much tighter control over the contract. Information had been a constant problem, but the Trust had now improved its internal methods and systems for data collection and reporting. It was still felt, however, that they were underresourced for this. Nevertheless, there was no explicit disagreement about problems with information at subsequent meetings between purchaser and provider, until the series of contract negotiation meetings in early 1995.

At those meetings, provider managers gave warnings about the need to clarify information about activity, particularly to adjust figures on patient contacts. An apparent fall in contacts was explained as the result of rising patient dependency (district nurses spent longer with fewer patients). The purchaser director of contracting accepted this possible explanation, but reminded the Trust representatives that their concern was with efficiency and effectiveness, so the Trust must *demonstrate* the increase in dependency: 'Information on this puts us *both* in a much stronger position.' Once more the providers referred to long-standing problems in their information system and asked for financial assistance from the health authority. Purchaser managers gave no commitment, but significantly, the director of contracting said he wanted to move away from the routine statistics:

> 'We need to focus on *health*, not these 'process' things. I want to contract for health and care, rather than tracking FCEs [finished consultant episodes] or whatever.'

In the event, Department of Health demands for purchasers to meet prescribed efficiency targets dominated their approach to information and monitoring. At the next negotiation meeting, purchaser and provider managers sought to find ways of meeting those targets without falling into the 'efficiency trap', i.e. if output or activity had been shown to increase beyond the target, then next year's baseline would be raised without commensurate increases in resources. The provider's suggestions for avoiding this trap were agreed. However, this agreement was then followed by a complaint by the Trust about the amount and frequency of requests for information by different health authority staff and by criticism of confusion within the purchaser organization about responsibilities for monitoring. Trust managers resented being asked to supply information for different purposes to several different sections within the purchaser. They also observed that there had been problems where variations in the contract had been informally agreed, but not documented, and then payments were delayed or not received. The Trust director of contracting insisted: 'We want a *formalized* contract monitoring process . . . We want complete documentation.' Purchaser representatives acknowledged that there might have been some internal confusion, caused by health-authority reorganization, and agreed to consider better coordination.

Occasionally, there were separate discussions during contract negotiations about the practicality of the purchaser's 'quality' specifications. The Trust argued that the quality section of the contract was unrealistic: *Patient's Charter* standards could not be completely met unless there was significant investment in Trust properties (for example, signposting, multilingual notices, improved facilities for disabled clients at clinic premises). The Trust claimed that the purchaser's standards could not be achieved in less than two years, and in any case, might not be worthwhile. Money spent on these aspects would have to be diverted from mainstream services. A more general point about the purchaser's demands was stressed by the provider director of contracting:

> 'None of it is costed. If there is monitoring on this, you must measure us on *realistic* standards . . . Some standards are more important than others. We're expected to sample survey four times a year on something we know we're not achieving and can't achieve. It's too much bureaucracy, and we'll spend hours and hours chasing our tails.'

While emphasizing that monitoring functions were crucial elements in the contract, the purchaser director of contracting accepted the Trust's argument and agreed a form of words which comprised a compromise position, phrasing the contract so that it referred to 'attainable' targets and priorities, and allowing for further joint discussion.

In the final round of interviews (in May 1995), the Trust director of contracting argued that while the amount of monitoring was not excessive, the very nature of community services makes it more difficult to quantify and measure effectiveness. The Trust chief executive believed that some community services could be measured, so they should begin with those and get better data. However, it was felt that purchaser managers did not have any insight into community services work, but at the same time they tried to get involved in operational matters under the cloak of monitoring. This was regarded as inappropriate and intrusive: 'They should be concentrating on outcomes, and the process (provided the quality of service is good) really should not be their concern – but they do try to get involved.' If penalties or incentives were applied in the contract, this must be on the basis of an agreed common currency and the targets must be 'reasonable and attainable'.

From the purchasers' perspective, the difficulties of measuring effectiveness were not seen as especially problematic in community services, though they were regarded as more severe in CHS and mental health services compared to acute hospital care. The purchaser director of contracting believed that it was feasible to develop outcome indicators for CHS (for example, leg ulcer recovery rates from treatment at home compared to hospital) and that kind of approach should be built in to the contract:

> 'A quarter of a million district nurse contacts tells me nothing; I don't think it tells the district nurses. The argument . . . is – if you've got a million pounds to invest, where can you get the most health gain?'

As part of this, monitoring had to be made more meaningful, related to quality and *Patient's Charter* standards as well as outcome indicators. This director of contracting stressed that the purchaser's demands for accountability were entirely legitimate. Similar views were expressed by the director of performance management. He thought that the problem of monitoring CHS was worse than that for acute hospitals, mainly because the information system was not very reliable and the units of information were meaningless (community contacts lasting two minutes or two hours were counted as identical). He believed that measuring effectiveness was *not* more difficult than in acute services and that greater commitment was required: the providers 'still hark back to the old wheeling and dealing arrangements with heartfelt arguments but without justifying effectiveness'.

Area 2

Compared with Area 1, in Area 2 purchaser–provider relationships were relatively more conflictual, and disputes about monitoring and information were recurrent issues during both contracting rounds. Once more, quality issues were not treated as separate concerns: arguments about monitoring necessarily focused on activity, resources and quality as interrelated elements.

Draft contract specifications drawn up by the provider in January 1993 described the composition of community services, outlined their mission statement and gave broad objectives for each service, acknowledging that national *Patient's Charter* and purchasing plan objectives would be pursued. There were no explicit references to outcomes or to quality assurance mechanisms. Following discussions with the purchaser, the next draft did contain a separate section dealing with 'quality assurance specification'. The contract stipulated that the Trust and the purchaser would 'work towards a programme of continuous quality improvement'; the Trust was expected to 'develop methods of measuring quality standards specified . . . in the contract' and 'work towards' agreed improvement targets. If these were not achieved, then there would be discussion to agree 'corrective action as appropriate'. The Trust and purchaser agreed to 'work together to develop a positive relationship for monitoring'.

During the contract negotiations in early 1993, Trust managers objected to the amount of detailed information (for example, on staff grades and numbers) demanded by the health authority. Purchaser representatives said they needed to check staffing against activity levels, but this caused disagreement during the meeting and tension afterwards. Within the Trust, this difference in approach to information was quite marked. According to key informants, the Trust opposed the type as well as the amount of information required by the purchaser. This information was regarded as a provider concern, Trust business. They were prepared to cooperate in working out some aspects of quality indicators, but the 'big issue' was how productivity and efficiency gain should be measured. Internally, and in meetings with the purchaser, Trust managers argued that the increasingly detailed monitoring of quality was inappropriate. Inside the purchaser, managers believed that the Trust possessed the information but was reluctant to disclose it to them: purchasers were determined to change this.

Later in the year, the Trust was still objecting to purchaser monitoring arrangements, arguing that they were inappropriate given the very recent reorganization of community services and the enlargement of the Trust. This issue surfaced repeatedly in purchaser–provider meetings. Trust managers said that they had insufficient staff and resources to provide the information requested by the purchaser, so they were looking for additional funding. This affected other aspects of the contract too, since they were unable to check apparent variances on activity levels and could not document their claim of increased workloads.

For the purchaser quality manager, the main concern was how to devise appropriate measures of effectiveness for CHS. He did not think that this was especially problematic, because they could develop professional standards for different specialties and also encourage the adoption of quality assurance procedures and management structures in the provider. The director of community care held similar views. He believed that although it was hard to identify the outcomes of district nursing or health visiting because their interventions are complex and the effects may be long term and not immediately obvious, it was possible to devise measurements of outcomes. The main reason it was slow to emerge, he argued, was that there was not yet a competitive market for CHS, information technology was inadequate, and the contracting culture had not permeated into community services in the same way as hospital services.

The health authority's 1993 purchasing plan contained numerous references to quality issues and the need to move towards a more explicit policy of commissioning health care with specified outcomes and health gains. The importance of the national *Patient's Charter* was underlined, and local objectives were indicated. The purchaser stressed that it was demanding improvements in services and required provider organizations to operate systems of quality assurance. It was noted, however, that it was not yet feasible to specify outcome measures for many of their priority objectives. Nevertheless, the health authority endorsed a 'partnership' approach with all providers to develop 'quality management systems' within the Trusts. Statements in the purchasing plan drew attention to particular national *Patient's Charter* standards which had to be met mainly in hospital services.

However, the plan also announced that the health authority intended to set targets in a number of community health services in order to improve the quality element of the contract. District nursing, health visiting, chiropody, speech therapy and community dental services were required to develop quality standards and quality management systems. The purchaser anticipated doing this through contract negotiations and by negotiation with the relevant provider professionals. The starting point for this was a belief that 'in order to maintain a partnership approach to purchasing it is essential to negotiate improvements in performance on the basis of providers' actual compliance with contractual standards and identify realistic, achievable increments'.

At the purchaser–provider contracting meetings in late 1993, the Trust expressed their anger at the 'tone' of some of the purchaser's proposals about quality requirements, arguing that they were more relevant to hospitals than community services. In response, the purchasers suggested that the Trust needed to have a better and stronger management of quality: as one manager put it: 'We're not convinced you've got that management in place. It needs to be strengthened.' The providers replied that they had not been resourced for this work and criticized health authority managers for approaching Trust service heads directly to discuss quality issues, rather than coming through the senior managers. Some agreement was reached that, in future, there would be 'joint' work on the monitoring of quality and purchasers were content to receive *any* information that would help them assess quality.

Relationships were still rather strained throughout the 1994 contract negotiations, linked to disagreements about finance, and the debate about quality and information continued. Provider informants perceived the purchasers as being dogmatic, and asking for too much information, too detailed information, too often. Not only was it technically difficult to obtain much of the information, it was extremely costly in staff time and effort, increasing their administrative costs.

The health authority placed quality monitoring on the contracting agenda again in its 1994 purchasing plan. Once more, the purchasers reminded providers that they should ensure they had 'comprehensive' internal quality management systems and should 'demonstrate a commitment to improving services . . . by assessing services against standards and targets'. In particular, they wished to extend the previous quality specifications to require providers to recognize the needs of carers of patients, clients with special needs and needs of ethnic minority groups. Most importantly for CHS, the purchasing plan demanded 'clearer accountability for services and value for money in these services'. Nine services were identified as requiring more detailed specification and quantification before the next contract was finalized.

Purchaser–provider meetings in 1994 were preoccupied with financial problems (as Chapter 6 showed), but disputes over information were closely connected with this wider debate. Purchasers asked repeatedly for the Trust to *share* information on activity levels, staffing and costs, as part of the discussion about the impact of service reductions. The Trust managers stressed that staffing and technical problems, exacerbated by the effects of recent amalgamation of units, made it impossible to supply the information demanded. This led to considerable annoyance and frustration within the health authority. As one senior purchaser manager expressed it: 'Unless we have the information, we can't fulfil our responsibility to improve health care – we'll feel powerless otherwise.' He felt that the providers were being uncooperative, and were unlike other Trusts in being so obstructive.

The series of continuing purchaser–provider meetings which led into negotiations about the 1995 contract were largely concerned with financial problems. However, there were frequent questions about whether the Trust was sharing relevant information with the health authority. As Chapter 6 shows, there were intense arguments about service reductions, and bargaining over service developments to be funded through greater cost efficiency, which all depended on the ability and willingness of the Trust to divulge detailed information about its business operations. Purchaser managers felt that the Trust was withholding important information, whereas the Trust managers believed that the purchasers' demands were excessive and intrusive.

Quality specifications had been successfully negotiated with all the major providers except for the CHS Trust. Internal briefing notes (prepared by the director of purchasing) for contract negotiations noted that, although a comprehensive quality specification for CHS had not yet been developed (because of the absence of community-based outcome measures and inadequate information systems), a request had been made to the Trust to consider proposals for the next contract. In a paper presented by the purchaser to a 'strategic liaison group' meeting with the Trust in December 1994, detailed demands were made, with specific objectives related to the volume and quality of services required, and 'key targets' identified to secure changes and improvements. These demands reflected the purchaser's disappointment and frustration that they had not made as much progress on CHS monitoring in general and quality in particular. For one key informant, monitoring was vital to contracting, but it was:

> '. . . essentially about the sharing of information, interpretation, the understanding of information, to see whether certain objectives have been reached, been achieved, been delivered. I think that if you have shared information, a shared understanding, you really will build a closer working relationship . . .'

For this purchasing manager, it was also important to do much more work on the effectiveness of CHS. Measuring the outcomes of community services was not regarded as being more difficult than hospital services. The main problem was the lack of a reliable information system. Another purchaser manager echoed these views, stressing that it was possible to measure some aspects of the effectiveness of community nursing, for example. Other purchaser respondents shared these managers' perception that the Trust had been reluctant to share information and had exaggerated the difficulties of quality monitoring. However, they were aware that outside of the formal negotiating machinery and senior management meetings, there were joint purchaser–provider working groups of middle managers who appeared to be trying to find practical solutions to these problems and there was a recognition of the necessity for collaborative working.

Within the Trust, by mid-1995, senior Trust managers still regarded monitoring as creating problems for them. There was an acceptance that they had to consider ways of demonstrating effectiveness, but a firm belief that the outcomes of community health services were intrinsically difficult to measure. As one interview respondent said:

> 'It's a great deal easier when you're producing nuts and washers, isn't it? When you are trying to improve somebody's well-being in the community, and improving the quality of their life – these things are difficult to measure, there is no doubt about that.'

Another senior provider manager also emphasized that community services are not easily identifiable and measurable, compared with hospital treatments. Certain community services (for example, physiotherapy) could define their outcomes easily, whereas health visiting was more nebulous; district nursing was probably intermediate between these. Monitoring, in principle, was acceptable but in practice it had to be appropriate and realistic. Hitherto, the purchaser was seen as pursuing inappropriate quality indicators, but now there were joint purchaser–provider specialist working teams trying to design better criteria and methods for monitoring and this was regarded as the most practical way to proceed.

After the signing of the 1995 contract, discussions continued outside of the formal contract negotiation machinery to agree more detailed and extended specifications for health promotion, family planning services and district nursing. The final draft documents included detailed schedules listing the composition of services, the information required by the purchaser (and its frequency), quality standards and monitoring procedures. The purchaser's general quality standards were supplemented by additional service-specific ones, although it was acknowledged, for example, that in health promotion 'routine monitoring arrangements do not easily apply'. The district nursing service specification contained a nine-page breakdown of objectives, listing standards and objectives, linking these with monitoring procedures. These included, for example: each patient to have an agreed appointment time within a two-hour period, with cards left with patients to record visits; 80 per cent of all visits to be by appointment; and quarterly data collection and occasional patient satisfaction surveys to check these arrangements were working. At a more clinical level, all patient care was required to be based on protocols and research-based practice; such protocols were to be established over time, and would be monitored by audits and through the development of outcome indicators. Clearly, these specifications reflected the purchaser's determination to establish a more systematic approach to monitoring and performance evaluation.

Thus there were different perspectives on the function and the feasibility of monitoring procedures and requirements. Compared with Area 1, the practicalities of information gathering and contract monitoring had generated much more explicit debate (and some disagreement) in Area 2. Discussions of quality, and about monitoring in general, were inevitably influenced by wider disagreement about resources and tensions in the purchaser–provider relationship. For purchasers, their main concern in monitoring was accountability; for providers, there were reservations about the feasibility and meaningfulness of such monitoring, given the particular characteristics of community services and inherent measurement problems.

Area 3

The HA purchaser in this area had taken a high public profile about its commissioning role, and stressed the importance of obtaining improvements in health gain, linked to specific targets from the *Health of the Nation* goals. It had experimented with various forms of devolved purchasing and promoted 'health alliances' with various agencies. Its 1993–4 purchasing plan noted that, to date, they had not influenced their major providers sufficiently, but that they intended to remedy this through a concerted strategy and explicit targeting of objectives in contracts. Community and primary care services were expected to become increasingly important, and CHS were given a high priority for resources.

The 1994–5 purchasing plan indicated that requirements for quality assurance by providers was based on a 'total quality management' (TQM) approach, linked to *Patient's Charter* and local quality objectives. Providers were expected to demonstrate that their organization met these TQM requirements. Clear statements of intention were also given to obtain improvements in certain services including primary-care nursing. These included clarifying the relationship between health visitors, district nurses, GPs and practice nurses, and set out various criteria for judging improvement. Later sections of the purchasing plan noted that the health authority intended to move towards more complex contracts with higher degrees of service specification and incentives to improve outcomes of service provision. The purchasers wanted to devise and agree quality indicators in each contract, and include 'milestones' to monitor the progress towards achieving local strategic goals.

Of course, in order to implement such plans, providers had to be persuaded and reliable information systems were necessary. Neither was entirely straightforward in community health services. The provider recognized from its inception as a Trust that information systems were inadequate. They were especially concerned to improve their information base in order to consolidate and expand their GP fundholding market (which was much larger than in Areas 1 and 2) as well as deal with the health authority purchaser. However, there was an official and declared commitment to pursue a 'quality strategy' within the Trust. This was acknowledged in internal documents such as the Trust's 1993 'statement of strategic direction'. There it was emphasized that among the *strategic* issues facing the Trust, they must evaluate the effectiveness of their services, and develop more sophisticated targets for performance, quality and outcomes 'which may be particularly complex for community services'. Detailed corporate objectives and service-specific objectives were given in which improved health outcomes and health gain were the recurrent theme. One of the strategic objectives given for community services was 'to develop measures of effectiveness, service quality and outcome which can be used in the contracting process'. The Trust's business planning guidance (prepared in late 1993 to brief directorates when making their own business plans prior to contract negotiations) instructed service heads to include performance monitoring against standards, as 'increasingly purchasers are asking for quality contract information'.

The 1994 corporate business plan stressed that effectiveness and efficiency would be continuously evaluated and that health gain was the principal objective for all services. Each service had very detailed and specific 'key objectives' and these were placed within a strategic statement about quality. This listed national and local *Patient's Charter* standards, waiting times, audit methods, nursing standards, user satisfaction surveys, etc. and also announced the establishment of a quality steering group to coordinate work across directorates.

Clearly then, the Trust had signalled its intention to take quality and performance evaluation seriously, and endorsed the purchaser's commitment to linking contracts with outcomes. However, this convergence was not always visible in the process of contract negotiations and routine monitoring meetings. For example, the purchaser finance director was dissatisfied with CHS information generally, especially with a currency expressed in nursing contacts, and, with other purchaser representatives, pressed for more outcome-oriented contracts to be developed. During contract negotiations in early 1994, information and monitoring did not figure as major items for discussion, although there were other routine meetings where statistics on activity were debated. Inside the purchaser, staff involved in managing contracts referred to difficulties in combining activity and finance data, and in linking this to quality indicators, and they noted that CHS were especially problematic. The Director of Finance referred to the fact that health authority members would ask questions about value for money, and it was therefore necessary to have more sensitive contracts and better monitoring.

Subsequently, the contract negotiations were dominated by disputes about finance; monitoring issues seemed not to be particularly controversial. Later in 1994, there were regular purchaser–provider contract review meetings, but discussion of information and monitoring appeared to be regarded as 'technical' matters, and did not cause any obvious or significant tension, whereas (as Chapter 6 shows) debates about service specifications and larger issues of funding were very vigorous. In December 1994, at a regular 'contract review' meeting, the purchaser representatives informed the Trust that they intended to have a separate quality section in the contract, as well as quality items in the service specifications. The providers accepted this framework, and the issue did not re-emerge at subsequent purchaser–provider meetings.

This acceptance probably reflects the fact that inside the Trust there already was a quality management system comprising quality groups in each directorate, overseen by a steering group, and each service was required to undertake regular performance reviews. This system had been reaffirmed in the 1994–5 business planning guidance. Each of the main community services (district nursing, health visiting) carried out systematic, but *internal*, professional audits (including separate monitoring of work for GP fundholders) and produced reports evaluating their activities.

Virtually all the contract negotiation meetings in early 1995 were preoccupied with possible cost cutting exercises and the level of Trust efficiency savings, and debating the merits of selective purchaser investment in specified services. Only at a special meeting to consider provider bids for service developments was there an explicit reference to problems of outcome measurement. Purchasers stressed that if they did commit extra funds, then they would require evidence of improvements in the quality of service and value for money. Provider managers argued that there were special problems in demonstrating effectiveness in various aspects of community nursing. This was then taken up in a later meeting, at which Trust representatives admitted that they lacked hard data on need and on effectiveness. In reply, a purchaser manager noted:

'Simply to put £60 000 into district nursing isn't on. It isn't easy to get a handle on what we're spending it on. It's not that we don't want to invest in district nursing but we want to wait for the information before we decide.'

In practice, the service specification for community nursing on which the eventual contract was based comprised 15 pages of detailed requirements, including 16 items about quality and four particular items for audit and outcome measures. It was noted that 'the provider and purchaser will collaboratively develop further quality standards and outcome measures for community nursing services'. The health authority contract document stated that 'the provider and purchaser agree to attempt to constantly improve the quality of actual care, outcomes, administration and access for patients' and the Trust was obliged to compile and supply information on the outcomes and level of quality achieved. In addition to this, there was a separate quality specification running to 46 pages with extensive and detailed schedules listing quality assurance requirements, local quality standards, *Patient's Charter* standards, national and local standards, and arrangements for quality improvement.

Reviewing their experience of the last contracting round, a senior purchaser manager claimed that they were handicapped in their monitoring because of problems with the CHS information system, but in principle it was no more difficult to define and measure effectiveness than in acute secondary care. He believed that much more work was necessary to identify the outcomes of CHS, and for the Trust to demonstrate evidence of improvements in services. There were signs of this happening, but this was almost independent of the contracting process. This informant argued that contracting had actually impeded worthwhile joint work on aspects like quality indicators, because it had generated conflict primarily over finance and resources.

Significantly, within the Trust, there was no sign that providers regarded the purchasers as making excessive or unreasonable demands on them for monitoring and information. The main concern was the dubious relevance of the contract currency – based on nursing contacts, which did not reflect case complexity or time – and persistent problems with the information system itself. One respondent acknowledged that the Trust was not always certain of the activity baseline, but this did not seem to have been an issue for the purchaser. GP fundholders were seen as being more demanding, but had been satisfied with what the Trust supplied. This manager was, however, anxious that in the near future the purchaser might attempt to become more formal and legalistic on matters of contract compliance and anticipated difficulties if this happened. Overall, the purchasers did not seem to regard monitoring in general, and quality evaluation in particular, as especially onerous or contentious.

Thus compared with both Areas 1 and 2, the issues of information, monitoring and quality did not feature as prominent subjects for argument or dispute in Area 3. Whether this reflects a conscious decision on the part of the purchaser not to pursue it, or a pragmatic recognition that little further progress could be made, or whether it indicates the existence of a basic culture of trust in the professionals delivering the service, is not clear. It may be a combination of these factors, but can also be explained as the consequence of other, largely financial issues dominating the contracting process. It is also arguable that, especially compared with the two other case-study providers, the Trust in Area 3 had a much more sophisticated and extensively developed 'infrastructure' for quality management, and made this very visible in its relationship with both the health authority purchaser and GP fundholders. This gave an assurance that they took these issues seriously and pre-empted a possible source of conflict in contract negotiations.

Conclusions

Comparing the three case-study areas, it can be concluded that there were important differences in the approaches taken by both purchasers and providers. All three health authorities had adopted a commissioning stance in which increasing emphasis was being given to contracting for outcomes and health gain. While all providers accepted these principles, the extent to which they embraced them, or were capable of adopting them, varied. These differences can be partly explained in terms of the structure and composition of the provider Trusts themselves and whether they had developed their internal quality management systems. Only in Area 3 was there a highly formalized system and set of procedures throughout the provider organization designed to deal with quality management. Significantly perhaps, this Trust in Area 3 was a very large unit which combined CHS with hospital-based maternity, children's and elderly services, where (it can be argued) methods for clinical audit and evaluation were already more advanced and well established. By contrast, the provider in Area 1 was much smaller in scale, and in Area 2 the provider had undergone major restructuring and amalgamation with other units. Both had comparatively less well-developed management systems for quality.

In addition to these organizational factors, however, there were also differences in attitudes concerning the degree to which providers were willing to comply with purchasers' demands for evaluation of performance and effectiveness. These were mainly influenced by the overwhelming importance of financial constraints and negotiations about activity, efficiency and resources, but they also indicated broader variations in purchaser–provider relationships, as indicated in Chapters 2 and 3.

In Area 1, despite an expressed determination to devise outcome-related contracts, during the fieldwork period no such contracts in CHS had emerged. The main obstacle to this according to both the purchasers and providers was the lack of a reliable information system and inadequate measurements of effectiveness. While there was an agreement to continue joint work on these matters, the provider insisted that quality targets had to be attainable and 'reasonable', and carried an administrative and financial cost. Once again, quality could not be disentangled from resources.

In Area 2, as noted previously, relations between the purchaser and provider were more conflictual, and there were constant arguments about the extent and type of contract monitoring required by the health authority. The purchasers, despite their declaration of a 'partnership' approach, nonetheless believed that the Trust was uncooperative and even obstructive in withholding information, and also regarded the Trust's quality management system as underdeveloped. The Trust objected to the amount, type and frequency of information demanded by the purchaser. They argued that it was difficult to produce without extra investment in information systems, and they doubted the feasibility of constructing valid measurements of effectiveness in many CHS. At the end of the fieldwork period, the status of contract monitoring was that attempts were being made to do more joint work to resolve these differences alongside collaborative work on service specifications, but the basic differences of perception remained.

As already noted, Area 3 displayed perhaps the most sophisticated attempts to build in quality monitoring to their contract. During the two rounds of contract negotiations observed, there were no obvious disputes about the nature and extent of quality monitoring. Both purchaser and provider acknowledged that further progress was dependent on improving the information system and developing service-specific clinical standards and indicators of outcomes. This was seen to be primarily a technical issue, although as the research ended, the experience of the last round of negotiations had led Trust managers to question the integrity of the purchasers. In their view, the controversial conclusion to the financial settlement of the contract had altered their entire thinking about the purchaser, and this then spilled over into their approach to other aspects of the contractual relationship. The hitherto collaborative and convergent approach to quality and monitoring had become threatened by arguments about resources.

Broadly, these findings appear to conform with those of other studies of NHS contracts (see NAHAT 1994). For example, in a detailed analysis of 118 contracts, Spurgeon and Smith (1995) found that there was poor specification of monitoring procedures and an acceptance among purchasers of an 'incremental' approach towards the development of quality standards throughout the term of a contract. Purchaser inspection visits and formal monitoring reports by providers seemed to be the most prevalent form of monitoring, but the recurrent emphasis was on working together. It was also noted that the majority of references to monitoring concerned activity and expenditure rather than service quality as such. Overall, there was a trend towards much greater formality in the language, organization and content of contracts (Smith 1994). However, in an analysis of GP fundholder contracts, Allen (1995) found that specifications for the monitoring of performance were 'deficient' and vague, outcomes were rarely mentioned and very few described methods of enforcement.

Of course, the capacity for regulation of quality depends very much on the nature of the service and the structure of the market. As Challis *et al.* (1994) have argued, in the NHS there are both concentrated purchasers and concentrated providers, so contracts are the 'natural instrument' for controlling standards, rather than external regulatory bodies. But as the number and complexity of contracts increases for any single purchaser (or provider), the problems and costs of monitoring become worse. Moreover, the nature of the service itself also places constraints on the possibility and type of monitoring. Knapp *et al.* (1994) and Wistow *et al.* (1994) point out that social care is 'different' from most other forms of personal and welfare service, and it is extremely difficult to define and measure quality in contracts. Consequently, a balance has to be struck, or trade-offs made, in the pursuit of 'tight' and 'loose' specifications.

It can be argued that this description of the special features of social care is very similar to CHS. There too, in making trade-offs about quality and monitoring, purchasers select a number of strategies, some or all of which may be adopted concurrently, as the case studies above show. Walsh (1995) suggested that where it is difficult to specify the work to be done and to monitor service performance, purchasers can introduce methods to ensure that their providers' commitments are credible (for example, performance bonds and quality assurance). Alternatively, they can try to ensure that providers share the same values as the purchaser, so that they are committed to delivering the service required (adopting identical mission statements and quality targets). Finally, they can deter failure through penal sanctions (deducting payments). Relationships of trust are more likely to be emphasized in contracts in which the service is more difficult to specify and sanctions are less likely to be invoked. The qualitative data from the case studies support this general argument and illustrate the particular problems of negotiating contract performance and quality in CHS. They also reveal the precarious nature of trust and the oscillation between assumptions about 'high trust/high discretion' relationships and 'low trust/low discretion' contracts (Fox 1974) in the internal market. This is discussed more fully in Chapter 8.

8

Markets, networks

and trust

The case-study evidence presented in the previous chapters illustrates the uneven and incomplete evolution of contracting in the internal market system within one sector of the NHS. It shows how different agencies responded to the complexity and difficulties of adopting an entirely new system founded upon notions of competitive bargaining for the supply of CHS.

It was shown in Chapters 1 and 2 that one of the most fundamental procedures – defining the content of community services in contract specifications – created considerable difficulties for most purchasers and providers. However, there were significant variations in the approaches adopted in each of the three areas. Both the health authority and the Trust in Area 1 saw the development of improved specifications as a joint exercise requiring collaboration, and this connected with the purchaser's preference for a relational or partnership style of contracting. In Area 2, in contrast, the health authority was much more adversarial in its demands about specifying the services required, although they professed a desire for a joint, shared approach. Progress in refining the specifications was slow and contentious. The purchaser and the provider in Area 3 each expressed the need for a collaborative approach to designing specifications. The health commission was determined to make services focus upon health gain and outcomes, and while the Trust were willing to adopt this philosophy, they were sceptical about its realism, and the eventual contract specifications remained general.

Some of these differences were also evident in relation to monitoring and regulation, discussed in Chapter 7. The purchasers in Area 1 were concerned to maximize health gain and were anxious to assess how well contracts 'delivered'. Health authority contract managers were keen to employ a partnership approach with the CHS provider, but meetings and formal negotiations were frequently dogged by arguments about the amount and validity of information. The providers resented what they regarded as the growth of excessive bureaucracy, the administrative costs they bore and the impracticality of some of the purchaser's quality standards.

There were also disputes about monitoring, as shown previously, in Area 2. The purchaser was predominantly concerned with accountability in terms of cost-efficiency and effectiveness, but also believed that the Trust had not developed its quality management system sufficiently. Purchaser managers often appealed to the Trust to share information with them but the provider managers reiterated that much of the information requested was unavailable, too costly to collect or collate and was methodologically questionable, particularly about outcomes. Informal working groups of managers attempted to resolve some of these problems, but they remained contentious matters. This was not the case in Area 3, however, where there were was a common commitment to the management of quality and a shared orientation to assessing the outcomes of services. Overall there was a consensual and pragmatic approach to monitoring, but this was disturbed by financial disagreements and the provider's lack of trust in the purchaser's commitments over resources.

As Chapter 6 also demonstrates, contract negotiations in all three areas were overwhelmingly concerned with finance and meeting activity and cost efficiency targets. Over the two contracting rounds observed, providers became increasingly aggrieved and distrustful about their treatment by the health authority purchasers. In Area 1, there were eventually broad agreements and compromises, but in 1995 this was qualified by provider resentment at what they regarded as inequitable treatment of community health services. There were major disputes in Area 2 in both rounds, with regional arbitration in 1994 and a struggle resulting in a very reluctant compromise between both parties in 1995. The purchasers viewed the Trust as uncooperative and intransigent, whereas the providers objected to the health authority's adversarial and dogmatic style, and their perceived failure to acknowledge the distinctive attributes and needs of CHS.

Similarly, in Area 3, despite rhetorical appeals to collaborative working, there were disputes over finance in both contract rounds, which were only settled through fiat by the respective chief executives outside of the formal negotiating team. The health authority adopted an assertive and 'robust' approach towards its contracts, and the Trust became increasingly suspicious and critical of its motives and actions, even to the extent of not trusting them on *any* issue.

In all three case-study areas, there were movements between apparently 'hard' and 'soft' approaches to contracting by the purchasers, and explicit attempts to develop a collaborative style of joint working at different times and over some issues. In general, however, from the providers' perspective, the regular appeal to develop 'shared understandings' was contradicted by purchasers' failure to commit sufficient resources and by intrusive and inappropriate forms of monitoring. The experience of contracting was one in which health authority purchasers implemented a 'low-trust' strategy, often evoking resentment and disillusionment among the providers.

Interestingly, this experience was *not* replicated in providers' dealings with GPs and GP fundholders, as Chapter 5 shows. The majority of GPs and GP fundholders placed a very high value on their local CHS and stressed their trust in the nursing professionals and the quality of their work. Contracting had enabled them to obtain improvements in information and to increase or modify particular services, but was not seen as a device to abandon current suppliers or even to coerce providers into changes. While there were some examples of 'adversarial' attitudes among some of the GP fundholders, they avoided bureaucratic or punitive styles of contracting in favour of much looser and more informal approaches. The possible threat of replacement by competitors from outside the locality was not seen as feasible or reasonable by most GPs and GP fundholders; instead, they appeared to endorse a network approach in which loyalty to colleagues in the primary health-care team – and appreciation of their local knowledge – was essential.

Reviewing the qualitative data, three aspects of the case studies are especially important. The first is that in each of the three areas, the particularity of CHS (their heterogeneity, their locality boundedness and the indeterminacy of their outcomes) presented fundamental problems for commissioning and contracting. The second point is that health authorities/commissions varied in the degree to which they adopted bureaucratic as against negotiative approaches to specifications and monitoring, and also varied in the extent to which they pursued adversarial or collaborative strategies in their contract negotiations. Some of this variation is due to differences in the purchasers' financial positions (and the severity of budget constraints), the legacy of previous investments in resources and services, and the emergent patterns of personal and interorganizational relationships following the purchaser–provider split.

We argue, however, that much of the variation can also be explained in terms of a third related feature apparent in the study – differential perceptions rooted in varying levels of trust. It was evident that for different groups within and between agencies (including GP fundholders), their commissioning and contracting behaviour was significantly influenced by their willingness to trust the other party in a whole range of circumstances. This finding is neither surprising nor controversial. Nonetheless, its importance and relevance derives from two more basic points. First, we argue that CHS by their very nature are extremely difficult to specify, 'contractualize' and monitor, and are also highly dependent on interprofessional and interagency collaboration. They thus require substantial amounts of trust in the professional discretion of providers. Second, the evidence from the three areas suggests that the actual *experience* of contracting, especially where assertive purchasers adopt 'hard' contractual styles, often engenders or exacerbates suspicious attitudes and feelings of mutual distrust. The first issue raises questions about the appropriateness and efficacy of competitive market contracting for a crucial component in the health care system. The second poses questions about the potentially corrosive effects of market relations and commodity exchange values on professional networks which depend on cooperation, reciprocity and interdependency.

It may be, of course, that the patterns of belief and behaviour described above are peculiar to the case studies and to the distinctive attributes of CHS. The indications from other studies (National Audit Office 1995; Rea 1995; Spurgeon and Smith 1995; Walsh 1995), however, suggest that they form part of a broader set of trends in the NHS internal market, and that CHS occupy an extreme point on a continuum of difficulty in contracting. This then provokes more fundamental questions about the kind of market being constructed within the NHS and the form of managed competition being practised. Findings from the case studies reported in previous chapters, and other studies, point towards contradictory and inconsistent policies which themselves reflect competing discourses about the operation of the market.

There are many different notions of what markets entail, and in the NHS these are invoked in different ways for different purposes at national and local level. One dominant and recurrent version appears to lay emphasis on a purchaser-driven market in which provider competition is stimulated to increase value for money and efficiency. Simultaneously, health authorities and Trusts are also exhorted to work collaboratively in conjunction with 'health alliances' towards joint goals. The annual contracting system is built on short-term calculations about activity and costs, but accomplishing changes in services and improving health gain outcomes involves long-term commitments. Central strategic objectives create pressures for purchasers to increase the volume of activity while controlling (or reducing) providers' costs *and* assume that purchasers and providers will cooperate in harmonious partnerships. Contract negotiations are the arena in which these potentially incompatible objectives are struggled over. Moreover, it is uncertain how far market contracts are congruent with, and are capable of sustaining, the networks and trust which are the defining attributes of, and prerequisites for, professional health-service delivery. In order to explore the reasons for this uncertainty further, we must discuss some of the crucial elements of the relationship between markets, networks and trust.

Markets

It is widely recognized that there are many different types of market, and that very few conform to the neoclassical image of perfect competition, with multiple buyers and sellers having complete information, motivated by utility (or profit) maximization, and supply and demand regulated by price. Most theoretical approaches in economics view markets as essentially allocative and coordinating mechanisms (Levacic 1993) for determining what to produce, how it should be produced and for whom. Market exchanges and transactions are mediated through voluntary contracts, and for contracts to be efficient there must be genuine competition (or contestability) and real incentives. These theoretical assumptions have been very influential in the creation of the NHS internal market, and indeed it has been argued that they have given rise to an inappropriate model of contracting predicated on ideas about individual bargaining (Mackintosh 1993). While the NHS is a managed market, its central presuppositions nonetheless endorse the virtues of competitive market contracts (Appleby *et al.* 1990; Jackson 1994). As Harden (1992) noted, consumer sovereignty was substituted by the separation of purchasers and providers, and competition was assumed to be inherent in their contractual relationship, which was founded on different interests and functions.

It is, however, also the case that the discourse of markets – whether 'real' or quasi' – contains many conceptual variants of markets, competition and contracts which often reflect abstract ideal types and normative assumptions rather than empirical reality. Williamson (1983, 1985, 1991) has cogently demonstrated that in business and industry, contracts and markets are only *one* form of coordination, and that transaction costs may make hierarchy (or vertical integration) and other 'hybrid' forms of economic organization efficient and preferable. In a related and important sociological critique of conventional economic theory, Granovetter (1985) has argued that idealized notions of competition and markets mistakenly exaggerate the significance of calculative individualism, and neglect the fact that economic behaviour is *socially embedded.* Granovetter stresses that personal relations and social networks based on trust are vital to maintaining exchanges within and between firms. For Granovetter, economic action cannot be explained as the outcome of self-interested, atomized, individuals in competition but is socially constructed and regulated: individuals' actions are 'both facilitated and constrained by the structure and resources available in social networks in which they are embedded' (Granovetter 1992: 7). Consequently, attention must be focused on the dynamics of those relationships and the extent to which they generate trust and deter 'malfeasance'.

A similar approach has been taken by those who recognize the ubiquity of long-term cooperation between ostensibly competitor firms and organizations, and who have noted the prevalence of 'relational' contracting. Commenting on Japanese business organization, Dore (1983) observed that stable and long-term commercial exchanges between companies entailed complex relationships founded on goodwill and diffuse but real patterns of mutual obligation. The resulting system of 'relational' (or obligational) contracting means that risks are shared, opportunistic exploitation is shunned, legal formalism is avoided in favour of trust, and the parties constantly look towards continued future trading. Bradach and Eccles (1991) argue that Williamson's markets versus hierarchy paradigm erects a false dichotomy, but also observe that relational contracting is important and that in commerce there are different combinations of relationships based on authority, price and trust.

Similarly, Powell (1991) noted that many types of economic organization fit neither the market nor the hierarchy model but rather exemplify *network* structures and alliances built on reciprocity and trust. Through these networks, the benefits and burdens of exchanges are shared and there is mutual dependency. Moreover, as Ring and Van den Ven (1992) have shown, contractual governance can include diverse business forms including consortia, franchises, and partnerships where cooperation is essential. They point out that in addition to short-term bargaining and opportunistic transactions between competing firms, there is also 'recurrent contracting' (where there are repeated exchanges of assets but contracts are short term). Relational contracts are favoured where services are jointly developed, there are highly specific assets, undertakings cannot be fully specified in advance, and mechanisms are sought to preserve long-term relationships. Such relational contracting is also argued to be especially appropriate (and effective) where there is a common desire to invest in highly specialized assets and technological innovation and where continuous exchange of information is essential, secured through 'bilateral dependence' (Bolton *et al.* 1994).

Evidently markets and contracts can embrace different types of commercial exchange and do not necessarily presume exploitative, opportunistic and pre-datory behaviour governed by immediate profit maximization. Furthermore, there are compelling economic and sociological arguments which promote the merits of relational contracts and network organization rather than ruthless competition between autonomous firms. What, then, are the attributes and advantages of 'network' forms of economic governance?

Networks

First it is necessary to briefly consider the concept of social network, in order to appreciate its economic and organizational implications. The importance of social network both as a metaphor for describing patterns of interpersonal relationships and as a tool in social research was first established by social anthropology and later developed within sociology. Clyde Mitchell (1969) focused attention on the nature of multiple links between actors and their influence on people's beliefs and actions. Networks – extended chains of con-nections and linkages – enable both the flow of communications and the exchange of goods and services. Bott (1971) showed how the density and connectedness of kinship networks affected social interaction and values, and also indicated how the concept of network could be used to analyse relation-ships between any group or organization and its environment. Such ideas have now become commonplace and applied in many different contexts including the study of corporate decision-making and political power, and can be used by different theoretical approaches to examine both formal and informal so-cial structures (Scott 1991). More recent interest in networks has arisen out of the critique of the markets and hierarchies paradigm and also debate about the emergence of 'post-modern' organizations.

Granovetter (1985) argued that empirically grounded explanations of econ-omic behaviour must incorporate people's real, concrete social relations (and social networks) which underpin all social exchange. Criticizing Williamson's markets and hierarchies model, Granovetter stressed the embeddedness of social relations between firms and highlighted the importance of 'intermedi-ate' forms of organization and contractual relationship. Economic action is accomplished by and through actors in networks rather than by atomized individuals (Swedberg and Granovetter 1992). Similarly, Powell (1991) rejected the markets–hierarchies dichotomy and argued that market exchanges are often based on collaborative ventures in which companies have 'dense ties' and alliances. A network structure is often preferred to secure mutual reliance and support, especially where there is a need for trust in the reliability and quality of the product or service supplied. Networks, Powell argued, are valuable for the exchange of commodities whose value cannot be precisely determined, such as 'know-how' and other services which are not easily priced or traded through the market.

Other writers have also observed that network structures, rather than formal bureaucracy or competitive contracts, seem particularly useful in enterprises which depend upon technological innovation, where personal obligations, reciprocity, commitment and trust are crucial in maintaining reputations as well as cooperation (Lincoln 1990; Larson 1992). In the analysis of public policy implementation, numerous researchers have identified the role that networks play in promoting, facilitating or obstructing policy initiatives both within and outside of formal structures (for example, see Dunleavy 1981; Hjern and Porter 1981; Hardy *et al.* 1990; Reid 1995).

Clearly, the concept of networks has widespread relevance and connotes distinctive forms of collective action which do not appear to fit conventional economic categories. Heydebrand (1989) anticipated the growth of new types of organizational forms (consequent upon economic and cultural changes in post-industrial capitalism) which replace formal bureaucracy and rigidly specified work patterns by flexible network arrangements, which rest upon informal norms and a corporate culture based on loyalty and trust. Such features are said to be characteristic of 'post-modern' organizations which require highly specialized flexible production and constant innovation, and also depend on highly skilled autonomous workers (see Reed 1992).

There is, of course, criticism of the idea that networks and network forms of organization are necessarily beneficent and well intentioned. Networks are used for many purposes and have many effects. Organizational theorists in the political economy tradition have shown how actors located in interorganizational networks are often engaged in conflict over resources. Networks are the medium through which power and dependency are expressed, and therefore networks can be benign or belligerent, inter- as well as intra-organizationally (Cook 1977; Benson 1978; Morgan 1990). There has been criticism too of contemporary managerialist endorsements of networks and networking as an organizational principle. It has been argued, for example, that fashionable management theory advocating networks conceals and mystifies relations of domination within organizations, and exaggerates the autonomous and consensual character of 'post-modern' work (Knights *et al.* 1993; P. Thompson 1993). Thus, while networks are ubiquitous, they are capable of embodying, and mobilizing, many different values and interests.

Finally, it must be noted that while some theorists identify networks as *alternatives* to (neoclassical) market competition, others do not regard them as *sui generis*. Indeed some analysts of business and marketing behaviour have described elaborate network arrangements, and a minimal level of cooperation and trust, as essential for market competition. Thus, some markets are composed of competing networks which are engaged in a continuous struggle for resources, where relationships may be antagonistic (Thorelli 1990).

Therefore, while it is possible for markets, hierarchies and networks to coexist (and for some networks to be exclusionary, particularistic and sectarian), it is also correct to observe that the most salient values associated with networks (altruism, loyalty, solidarity, reciprocity, trust) are likely to influence social exchanges and contractual relationships in distinctive ways (G. Thompson 1993).

These values are exactly those that characterize 'clan' forms of social organization, which have also been argued to comprise alternative modes of economic coordination (Heydebrand 1989). Ouchi (1991) noted that the transaction costs necessary to validate market transactions as being equitable for contracting parties are frequently high, and that bureaucratic authority entails extensive surveillance and assumes goal congruence among organizational actors. Neither approach deals adequately with situations in which the criteria for performance evaluation are ambiguous and/or there are divergent goals. Instead, Ouchi suggested that *clans* offer the potential for cooperative and collective action, legitimized through common allegiance and socialization. Ouchi suggested that clans are particularly appropriate in technologically advanced industries and services requiring teamwork, and where an individual's task performance is inherently ambiguous (for example, in professional services). Clans monitor and evaluate behaviour through informal means and peer pressure, rather than through explicit audit and verification: 'there is sufficient information in a clan to promote learning and effective production, but that information cannot withstand the scrutiny of contractual relations' (Ouchi 1991: 252).

Some researchers have found that clan forms of social control are effective in industrial settings and can possess both an economic as well as a social-integrative function. Alvesson and Lindkvist (1993), for example, have distinguished between a corporate culture which may be based on opportunism and competition, and a clan structure in which members have a collectivistic and solidaristic orientation. Clan forms necessitate 'loose' or 'soft' modes of contracting, and Alvesson and Lindkvist found more empirical evidence of social integrative rather than economic clans.

There is thus a large body of theoretical and empirical work which suggests that there are special types of social structure (whether termed 'networks' or 'clans') which exhibit distinctive attributes, values and behaviour, and which are difficult to reconcile with either neoclassical notions of contracts and market competition or bureaucratic hierarchy. Central to all of this work is a convergence on the importance of trust and the management of risk in economic and social exchange.

Trust

All social interactions presuppose some minimal degree of trust, although expectations will vary according to the nature of the exchange. Giddens (1991) has noted that trust is essentially about confidence and reliability, but these are necessarily contingent on awareness of risk. One of the defining features of modern societies is the shift away from reliance on personalized trust towards dependency on trust in abstract systems. The former (experienced through interpersonal commitments) is never entirely displaced but is extended and subsumed in wider institutional trust and faith in expert knowledge, for example. Trust would not be necessary, as Giddens observed, if the other party's actions were constantly visible, if their motives were transparent and their activities fully understood. It is precisely contingency, uncertainty and lack of information which renders trust so necessary and so important. It is also those exigencies which makes it a continuous problem (or 'project') to be worked at.

This point has also been frequently stressed by other writers. Barber (1983) argued that trust was rarely completely accomplished in social relationships, and that maintaining it is a reciprocal and endless task. Similarly Luhmann (1979, 1988) emphasized that trust is a way of reducing complexity, is always related to risk, and must be both actively achieved and learned. However, that may be intrinsically difficult or precarious in certain types of social exchange. Barber (1983) argued that technically competent performances can be monitored if they are based on shared knowledge and expertise, but if some parties to a social relationship cannot understand that expertise, the performance can only be controlled by trust. Such trust may be insufficient in the case of professional work, where supplementary control mechanisms are required. Conversely, distrust may weaken the basic assumptions of confidence and cooperation needed for successful transactions to take place.

There is thus a complex dialectic of trust–distrust which affects all social relationships, but it is especially manifest in all forms of economic exchange and contractual behaviour. This fundamentally important issue was cogently analysed by Fox (1974) in ways which still have direct relevance and application. Fox, discussing the exercise of authority in workplace and employment relationships, argued that there were two distinct 'syndromes' of work roles based on different amounts of discretion, and that these corresponded with different amounts and forms of trust–distrust.

In a 'high-trust relationship,' participants:

- share (or have similar) ends and values;
- have a diffuse sense of long-term obligation;
- offer support without calculating the cost or expecting an immediate return;
- communicate freely and openly with one another;
- are prepared to trust the other and risk their own fortunes in the other party; and
- give the benefit of the doubt in relation to motives and goodwill if there are problems.

In contrast, in 'low-trust' relationships', participants:

- have divergent goals and interests;
- have explicit expectations which must be reciprocated through balanced exchanges;

- carefully calculate the costs and benefits of any concession made;
- restrict and screen communications in their own separate interests;
- attempt to minimize their dependence on the other's discretion; and
- are suspicious about mistakes or failures, attributing them to ill-will or default and invoke sanctions.

Fox argued that, increasingly, purely economic exchanges and those relying on formal contracts institutionalized the dynamics of low trust and low discretion. Social exchange, conversely, entails diffuse obligations, judgement in task performance, and loyalty, and requires and sustains high-trust relationships and high levels of work discretion. He claimed that in modern societies, the permeation of virtually every sector of social life by contractual and market relations had undermined the reciprocity and diffuse obligations which are necessary for high-trust relationships. Thus, 'The keen calculative specificity of reciprocation which characterises purely market transactions is a contradiction in terms to . . . high-discretion relations' (Fox 1974: 374).

We thus arrive back at the paradox or dilemma that, while high-discretion work (for example, complex professional services) may necessitate high levels of trust, this, as Granovetter (1985) observed, presents increased opportunities for malfeasance. Dogmatic attempts to codify, formalize and prescribe such high-discretion work will not only be infeasible but also counterproductive, because prescriptive contracts are inappropriate for tasks characterized by indeterminacy and uncertainty, and the use of sanctions (resting upon distrust) will undermine the contractual relationship. This dilemma, moreover, appears in recent approaches to contracting in the NHS quasi-market, and is evident in the case-study material discussed earlier.

Quasi-market contracts, networks and trust in community health services

In his review of contracting practice in the public sector, Walsh (1995) concluded that the nature of the service and product complexity determined the extent to which contracts could be formalized, limiting the degree to which they can be fully specified and monitored. He pointed out that in many health and social services, outcomes are difficult to define and performance is hard to measure, so a significant element of trust is required and inevitable. However, he also observed that the development of internal market contracts 'has the effect of leading to formalisation, duplication and pressure on trust-based relationships' (Walsh 1995: 161). He further argued (1995: 255) that:

> . . . the danger of contract is that it undermines trust through basing contracts on punishment for failure. If we undermine trust then we may find that the making of agreements, and ensuring that they are kept, will become very costly.

Walsh's assessment seems to be broadly confirmed by the case-study evidence presented earlier. Many of the difficulties encountered by purchasers and providers at each stage of the commissioning and contracting cycle derived from the complexity and diffuseness of CHS and these were compounded by fluctuations in the extent to which parties were prepared to trust each other. The imposition of quasi-market competition and purchaser-dominated contracting posed fundamental questions about the culture, structure and organization of community nursing and some of the other community-based therapy and specialist services.

Most provider chief executives, business managers and professional service managers were committed to expand and market their specialist skills, but were frequently perplexed by what they regarded as unrealistic and unnecessary purchaser demands for detailed specifications, continuous verification of statistical returns about activity, and requests for precise definitions of outcomes and quality. Purchaser insistence that providers demonstrate their value for money and effectiveness in relation to health gain, while acknowledged as predictable and legitimate concerns, nevertheless regularly prompted the response from providers that CHS were special and could not be easily identified or measured in ways that permitted unequivocal answers. The distinctive features of CHS (it was asserted) required high levels of trust and pragmatic understanding rather than formalized contracting. Implicitly, at least, there was a presumption of the intrinsic network attributes of community services, and an expectation among many provider staff (partly shared by some, but not all, purchasers) that 'soft' contracting and collaborative relations were not only desirable in themselves but also the only practicable approach.

The particular attributes of CHS have already been discussed in Chapters 1 and 2, but it is worth restating some of their core characteristics. The Audit Commission's *Homeward Bound* (1992a) indicated the increasing importance of CHS, and noted their complexity, their *network* character, their multi-disciplinary and multi-agency working, but also criticized their relative lack of integrated management. Smith *et al.* (1993) emphasized that district nursing work essentially comprises both clinical and networking skills, and is based on a 'holistic' view of patients' needs and health. They noted that much of community nurses' workload was invisible but that among their greatest assets were their detailed *local knowledge* of communities, neighbourhood health needs and the range of informal and formal sources of care. Mackintosh (1993: 150) observed:

> To sit in a health clinic and watch the networking between community nurses based there, other clinic staff, home care workers, Macmillan nurses and the public is to realise the density of the local information which passes through and to appreciate that such local knowledge is a joint product with nursing care.

Similarly, Lightfoot (1994) has noted that community nursing is characterized by being peripatetic (and thus difficult to supervise) and 'the nature of the work necessitates operating in a pragmatic way at the boundary between health and social care' (1994: 98).

Exworthy (1994) draws attention to the fact that CHS have disparate functions, that community nursing is delivered in many different settings, that most CHS embrace a 'social' rather than a 'medical' approach to health care, and that they have 'fluid' organizational boundaries with other professions and agencies (including GPs and local authority social services). Twigg and Atkin (1994) identify three main types of function performed by community nurses, and suggest that these are, again, specialized assets with high levels of public approval. Community nursing thus consists of:

- clinical treatment and care;
- personal or social care; and
- advocacy and gatekeeping in connection with referral to other agencies and services.

While they are undoubtedly at nodal points in the primary-care network (Øvretveit 1993), community nursing and other CHS professionals are also located in what Dalley (1991) refers to as an uncertain or 'uncontrolled' environment which is difficult to manage. It is precisely for these reasons that Øvretveit (1993) rejects market and bureaucratic modes of organization as inappropriate for CHS, in favour of what he terms 'associational' (or network) structures, underwritten by relationships of trust and shared values.

Collaboration and teamwork are thus regarded as intrinsic to, and necessary for, the practice of CHS. As the Audit Commission (1992a: 5) report on CHS noted:

Operating in concert with GPs, local authority social services, voluntary organisations, the private sector and unpaid carers, they are an essential element in the wider network that provides 'primary care'.

The report then referred to the flexibility of the community health workforce at the centre of this network, and the 'unique nature of this central role'. In the closely related sector of community care, the Audit Commission (1992b) also laid great stress on the need for coordination between local authority social services, health authorities and CHS providers, and other voluntary and private sector bodies. Legislative requirements and official guidance frequently refer to the necessity for collaboration and joint working, the aim being to achieve 'seamless care', so that clients or patients are not aware of organizational barriers between primary and community-based health care, secondary health care and social care.

In the internal market, however, there are structural constraints which limit the scope of, and incentives for, interagency collaboration and coordination. Øvretveit (1993) has extensively described some of the operational issues involved in the coordination of community health and social care and made practical suggestions for improvements. He has also, however, argued that neither market or bureaucratic modes of organization facilitate collaboration: coordination is more difficult to obtain where actors' interests and values are divergent and where they have different objectives. Associational or network approaches are proffered as most likely to secure more effective coordination, but these are weakened by the impact of market competition. As Øvretveit (1993: 202) notes:

More pressure on resources and 'market competition' can work against co-ordination, but co-ordination can save costs and agencies can often better achieve their goals through co-operation rather than through competition or isolation.

Even if there is some support for the principles of collaborative or network organization, there is a long established history of interprofessional rivalry and even conflict among NHS professions which may make coordination extremely difficult. Hugman (1995) has discussed the difficulties of interprofessional working, arguing that because the boundaries of health and social care are contested, this poses problems for the provision of seamless care. Some professions, he argues, are inward-looking and defensive of established practice, and this is a barrier to the flexibility demanded by the new market environment. Reviewing the joint commissioning function in health and social care, Hudson (1995) is sceptical about its feasibility. Analysing various modes of collaboration from networks through coalitions and federations to complete integration, Hudson nevertheless suggests that it is uncertain how (and whether) trust can be developed in interorganizational networks formerly noted for rivalry and mistrust. The quasi-market makes the task *more* problematic, according to Hudson (1995: 246):

> In general . . . there is some contradiction between the principles of collaborative working and collective responsibility and the fostering of a quasi-market based upon principles of competition and individual responsibility.

There are thus certain key elements of CHS organization and expertise, especially their decentralized autonomy, flexibility, network form and capacity for coordination, which gives them a pivotal role in primary care. But it is also those attributes which are potentially damaged by the rigid application of competitive market contracting.

Smith *et al.* (1993: 123) found that assertive purchasing, adopting 'tight' contract specifications was 'likely to undermine the joint production of local information, networking and nursing care necessary for a quality service'. In the same case study, Mackintosh and her colleagues (1993) found that contracting had eroded the sense of professionalism among community nurses. Purchasers' (and provider managers') demands to specify work content, skill and case mix in great detail, and constant monitoring of activity and an emphasis on rapid throughput were regarded with suspicion and some opposition by frontline staff. Mackintosh argued that quality control required the nurses' commitment and goodwill, but 'hard' contracting styles and tight specifications threatened that goodwill. She concluded (1993: 144):

> While one should not overpolarise . . . there *is* a conflict between a view emphasising close joint working and field staff involvement [in purchasing] and a view preferring arm's length relations with providers, purchaser initiative and tight contract specification.

In case studies of three CHS Trusts and community nursing by the Royal College of Nursing, it was found that community nurses placed the highest value on patient care, but saw this as being undermined by the financial and management work resulting from the internal market. 'Bureaucracy' was seen as colonizing the caring role and GP fundholding was also perceived as a significant encroachment on nurses' professional autonomy. The operation of the internal market had made collaboration among the primary health-care team more difficult. Moreover, measures to increase efficiency by altering skill mix, stimulated by contractual pressures, were perceived by community nurses as fragmenting their work and reflecting a failure to understand the holistic nature of nursing practice (Traynor and Wade 1994; Traynor 1995).

Similarly, Duggan (1995) refers to anxieties and uncertainties among community nursing staff about the impact of competition. On the one hand, there are opportunities for them to market their specialist skills and local knowledge (and there are expanded roles available especially for district nurses and health visitors) to different purchasers, but on the other hand efficiency-driven changes in skill mix may lead to 'de-skilling' and there are perceived threats to autonomy because of the prospect of direct management by GP fundholders.

In closely related areas of health care, there are very similar findings and predictions. In the field of palliative care where specialist community nurses' (such as Marie Curie and Macmillan nurses) and the voluntary sector hospices' role in the care of the terminally ill is increasingly important, Clark *et al* (1995) found that contracting was seen as creating problems. The need for joint purchasing strategies among health authorities and local authority social services, and for links with CHS and voluntary sector agencies, was put under strain by the market. Voluntary sector providers feared the loss of their independence, and the purchaser–provider split was seen as detrimental for the partnership necessary for organizing and delivering palliative care. In Rea's (1995) study of a large combined hospital and community mental health services Trust, there was widespread ambivalence among managers and professionals about competition and market-like behaviour. Moreover, Rea reported that *within* the Trust there were conflicts between the mental health directorate and the medical directorate about finance and other resources. These conflicts, and other market-driven pressures, undermined their declared strategy for developing community based mental health services.

It can thus be concluded that there is a significant body of diverse but relevant evidence which supports and amplifies the findings from the case-study research discussed in previous chapters. Community services are constituted in network forms and offer their network character as a distinctive advantage for the particular set of tasks that primary care requires. Professional discretion and flexibility, together with collaborative teamwork, are deemed to be both core values and organizational prerequisites for most community practitioners. Their clanlike structure, and their promotion of the virtues of cooperation and interdependence, necessitates both a management approach and a purchasing strategy based on high trust, and soft or relational contracting. However, as this book has shown, the quasi-market has evoked attitudes and behaviour among many purchasers which do not promote or facilitate such an approach. It remains to be seen whether future changes in the structure of purchasing, and modifications in the contracting system, will result in the acceptance of these distinctive features, or will seek to amend or even subvert them.

Appendix:
Methodology

The empirical findings reported in this book are derived from a three-year study (1992–5) funded by the Economic and Social Research Council, as part of its 'Contracts and Competition' research programme. The project was designed to gather information about the *process* and *experience* of contracting for CHS, and therefore adopted a case-study approach. In particular, because it was necessary to understand the perceptions and actions of a range of different CHS purchasers and providers, as well as representatives of patients and users, qualitative research methods were used in a limited number of sites.

The main advantage of qualitative methods is that they allow the researcher to understand the meaning of social action through intensive fieldwork over time, and provide an insight into actors' beliefs (and organizational cultures) as well as the local dynamics of change in their natural setting. The project therefore used *ethnographic* methods and a case-study design, using non-participant observation, unstructured and structured interviews, and the collection of documents (see Hammersley and Atkinson 1983; Hammersley 1990).

Observations of meetings were recorded and verbatim notes made of discussions *in situ*. The majority of structured interviews were tape-recorded and transcribed; in others, contemporary verbatim notes were made. Data were then analysed and interpreted using the principles of analytic induction and grounded theory, with methodological triangulation by comparison of findings from different sources and separate sites (see Rosen 1991; Bryman and Burgess 1994). All three authors were involved in the fieldwork, data analysis and interpretation, though each specialized in certain issues and themes. The intention was to produce a detailed understanding of the context within which contracts were defined, negotiated and monitored, to analyse the complex interrelationships between different NHS agencies, and to explore the views of clients. The data presented in this book represent an important contribution to what the late Phil Strong termed 'policy ethnography' (Strong and Robinson 1990: 8) and build on other qualitative studies of decision-making and policy implementation in the NHS (see Pettigrew 1990; Pollitt *et al.* 1990).

When the project was planned, it was decided that to examine the operation of the internal market and the effects of competitive contracting in CHS, it was necessary to undertake comparative analysis of experience in several areas, to concentrate within one NHS region in England to observe the possibility of local competition, and to carry out research over more than one 'round' of contracting. Budget and time constraints, as well as important access considerations, finally determined the selection of a sample of three fieldwork sites and the period of investigation (in two contracting cycles: 1993–4 and 1994–5).

Initially, two large contiguous metropolitan DHAs in one NHS region were chosen because they had different organizational structures and different approaches to commissioning and purchasing:

- **Area 1.** Here there was a single DHA and separate FHSA, but they had embarked on closer collaboration and joint 'commissioning for health gain'; there was also a directly managed community unit about to become a Trust.
- **Area 2.** Here there was a purchasing consortium representing three separate DHAs, and one FHSA for the whole area. CHS were provided by one large specialist community unit in one DHA, and by combined acute/community units in the two other districts. The specialist CHS unit became a Trust in 1993 and then assimilated the other community services from the nearby districts through amalgamation.

During the first phase of fieldwork, the DHAs in Areas 1 and 2 underwent 'reconfiguration' through mergers with other adjacent DHAs, and the initial differences in the formal organization of purchasing appeared to diminish. For this reason an additional site was included:

- **Area 3.** This was noted for having an integrated DHA/FHSA and a reputation for innovation in health commissioning. It also contained a very large Trust which comprised CHS linked with hospital-based directorates for children's, elderly and maternity services.

Given assurances about respecting confidential information and guaranteeing anonymity for the agencies and individuals, the purchaser and provider organizations in all the three areas agreed to allow us to carry out research. The way in which fieldwork is reported and interpreted thus reflects the necessity to maintain anonymity. Interviews were held at various stages of each contracting round with the chief executives, directors of finance, directors of contracting and other key managers (for example, those responsible for health needs assessment, monitoring, quality assurance) and selected medical professionals in each DHA. We regularly attended and observed meetings of purchaser specialist groups and officer teams which prepared the purchasing plan, coordinated public consultation, formulated purchasing and commissioning strategy and oversaw contract negotiations.

In the provider Trusts, interviews were held with the chief executives, the directors of contracting and corporate strategy, the directors of finance, the business and contracts managers, quality assurance managers, clinical directors, and the professional heads of community nursing and other therapy services. In addition, wherever possible, we attended senior management meetings at which contracting issues were debated. Most importantly, we were able to attend the formal contract *negotiation* meetings between the Trusts and the DHA purchasers, as well as their regular 'contract monitoring' and service commissioning meetings. In two districts, we were also fortunate to observe some of the contract negotiation meetings between the Trusts and local GP fundholders.

Copies of all relevant documents, at every stage of drafting, were obtained, including: contracts; purchasing plans; business plans; contract specifications and schedules; briefing notes for negotiation meetings; internal memoranda; correspondence between purchasers and providers; and the official minutes of most meetings. To gain some impression of the scale and value of contracts and activity involved, the areas comprised Trusts with community staff ranging from 750 to 1000 whole-time equivalent posts, dealing with community activity of about 500 000 to 700 000 patient contacts per year, with total DHA contract values from £13 million to £29 million per year in 1994–5.

Another important part of the project was to gather information about the involvement of patients or users in CHS contracting. Here, because of the heterogeneity of client groups, there was no reliable and readily identifiable 'sampling frame'. Instead, using local directories and other sources, contacts were made with a very large number of individuals and groups representing actual and potential clients of CHS (including the elderly, mentally ill, disabled and ethnic minority groups). The local community health councils, council for voluntary service and other voluntary sector organizations in each area, as well as the DHAs and Trusts, also supplied lists of client group representatives, and through 'snowballing', further contacts were made. Unstructured and semistructured interviews were then held with key informants (see Pickard *et al.* 1995).

While the bulk of the fieldwork was concerned with relationships between Trusts and their main purchasers (the DHAs) the research also tried to examine the impact of GP fundholding and the involvement of GPs in DHA purchasing. In the three areas, an initial pilot interview survey was carried out on a random sample of GPs and GP fundholders. In the spring and summer of 1994, structured (tape-recorded) interviews were held with a purposive sample of 10 GP fundholders, selected from the three areas; interviews were also held with a small number of GP fundholder practice and fund managers, as well as non-fundholding GPs. The final sample size was smaller than expected, owing to the relatively low rate of fundholding in the areas, and also because of doctors' reluctance to give up time to participate: some GPs and GP fundholders complained about being 'overresearched'. Nevertheless, the qualitative data obtained are valid, and based on the pilot survey and studies by other authors, appear reliable.

While the findings discussed in this book are not statistically representative of the national scene (precisely because they are derived from a case study using qualitative methods) it is, nonetheless, believed that the data are high in validity and are consistent with those from other research, and therefore reliable and capable of wider generalization. The interpretations of the data are, we believe, coherent and consistent, and broadly reflect the wider experience elsewhere of contracting for CHS during the period of fieldwork.

References

Acheson, R. (1988) *The Report of the Committee of Enquiry into the Public Health Function* (Acheson Report). London: HMSO.

ACHEW (1991) *GP Fund-holding: Profit or Loss for Patients?* London: Association of Community Health Councils.

ACHEW (1994) *Community Health Services*. London: Association of Community Health Councils for England and Wales.

Allen, P. (1995) Contracts in the National Health Service internal market, *Modern Law Review*, 58(3): 321–42.

Alvesson, M. and Lindkvist, L. (1993) Transaction costs, clans and corporate culture, *Journal of Management Studies*, 30(3): 427–52.

Appleby, J. (1994) The reformed National Health Service: a commentary, *Social Policy and Administration*, 28(4): 345–58.

Appleby, J., Little, V., Ranade, W., Robinson, R. and Smith, P. (1991) *Monitoring the White Paper: Managed Competition Project paper No 4*, Implementing the reforms – a national survey of district general managers. Birmingham: National Association of Health Authorities and Trusts.

Appleby, J., Little, V., Ranade, W., Robinson, R. and Smith, P. (1992) *Implementing the Reforms: A Second National Survey of DGMs*, NAHAT project paper 7. Birmingham: National Association of Health Authorities and Trusts.

Appleby, J., Robinson, R., Ranade, W., Little, V. and Salter, J. (1990) The use of markets in the health service: the NHS reforms and managed competition, *Public Money and Management*, Winter: 27–33.

Arnstein, S. R. (1969) A ladder of citizen participation in the USA, *Journal of the American Institute of Planners*, 35(4): 216–24

Audit Commission (1986) *Making a Reality of Community Care*. London: HMSO.

Audit Commission (1992a) *Homeward Bound*. London: HMSO.

Audit Commission (1992b) *Community Care – Managing the Cascade of Change*. London: HMSO.

Audit Commission (1993) *Their Health, Your Business*. London: HMSO.

Barber, B. (1983) *The Logic and Limits of Trust*. New Brunswick, NJ: Rutgers University Press.

Barker, G. (1992) GP fundholding: sold out to slow extinction, *Health Visitor*, 65(12): 455.

Barnes, M. and Wistow, G. (1992) Understanding user involvement, in M. Barnes and G. Wistow, *Researching User Involvement*. Leeds: Nuffield Institute for Health Services Studies, University of Leeds.

Barnes, M., Prior, D. and Thomas, N. (1990) Social Services, in N. Deakin and A. Wright (eds) *Consuming Public Services*. London: Routledge. pp. 105–53.

Bartlett, W. (1991) Quasi-markets and contracts, *Policy and Politics*, 11(3): 53–61.

Bartlett, W. and Le Grand, J. (1993) The theory of quasi-markets, in J. Le Grand and W. Bartlett (eds) *Quasi-Markets and Social Policy*. London: Macmillan.

Bartlett, W. and Harrison, L. (1993) Quasi-markets and the NHS reforms, in J. Le Grand and W. Bartlett (eds) *Quasi-Markets and Social Policy*. London: Macmillan.

Benson, J. K. (1978) The interorganizational network as a political economy, in L. Karpik (ed.) *Organization and Environment*. London: Sage.

Beresford, P. and Harding, T. (1993) *A Challenge to Change: Practical Issues of Building User-led Services*. London: National Institute for Social Work.

Bolton, M. K., Malmrose, R. and Ouchi, W. G. (1994) The organization of innovation in the United States and Japan – neoclassical and relational contracting, *Journal of Management Studies* 31(5): 653–79.

Bott, E. (1971) *Family and Social Network*, 2nd edn. London: Tavistock.

Bowling, A., Jacobson, B. and Southgate, L. (1993) 'Health service priorities', *Social Science and Medicine*, 37(7): 851–7.

Bradach, J. and Eccles, R. (1991) Price, authority and trust, in G. Thompson, J. Frances, R. Levacic and J. Mitchell (eds) *Markets, Hierarchies and Networks*. London: Sage.

Bryman, A. and Burgess, R. (1994) Developments in qualitative data analysis, in A. Bryman and R. Burgess (eds) *Analyzing Qualitative Data*. London: Routledge.

Calnan, M. and Gabe, J. (1991) Recent developments in general practice, in J. Gabe, M. Calnan and M. Bury (eds) *The Sociology of the Health Service*. London: Routledge.

Carruthers, I., Fillingham, D., Ham, C. and James, J. (1995) *Purchasing in the NHS: The Story So Far*. Health Services Management Centre discussion paper 34. Birmingham: Health Services Management Centre, Birmingham University.

Chalkley, M. and Malcomson, J. (1994) Contracts and Competition in the NHS. Paper presented to the ESRC Contracts and Competition Programme Conference, 19–20 September, Robinson College, Cambridge.

Challis, L., Day, P., Klein, R. and Scrivens, E. (1994) Managing quasi-markets: institutions of regulation, in W. Bartlett, C. Propper, D. Wilson and J. Le Grand (eds) *Quasi-Markets in the Welfare State*. Bristol: School for Advanced Urban Studies.

Clark, D., Neale, B. and Heather, P. (1995) Contracting for palliative care, *Social Science and Medicine*, 40(9): 1193–202.

Clyde Mitchell, J. (1969) The concept and use of social networks, in J. Clyde Mitchell (ed.) *Social Networks in Urban Situations*. Manchester: Manchester University Press.

Cook, K. (1977) Exchange and power in networks of interorganizational relations, in J. K. Benson (ed.) *Organizational Analysis*. London: Sage.

Cunningham, M. and Culligan, K. (1990) Competitiveness through networks of relationships in information technology product markets, in D. Ford (ed.) *Understanding Business Markets*. London: Academic Press.

Cutler, T. and Waine, B. (1994) *Managing the Welfare State*. Oxford: Berg.

Dalley, G. (1991) Patterns of management in community units, in A. McNaught (ed.) *Managing Community Health Services*. London: Chapman and Hall.

Dawson, D. (1994) *Costs and Prices in the Internal Market*, Centre for Health Economics, discussion paper 115. York: University of York.

Deakin, N. (1993a) A future for collectivism?, in R. Page and J. Baldock (eds) *Social Policy Review 5*. Canterbury: Social Policy Association.

Deakin, N. (1993b) Contracts and Competition in the Management of Public Services: A Comparative Study. Paper first presented to a conference at South Bank University.

Department of Health (1988) Circular (E(88)64). London: Department of Health.

Department of Health (1989a) *Working for Patients*, London: HMSO.

Department of Health (1989b) *Working for Patients: Contracts for Health Services – Operational Principles*. London: Department of Health.

Department of Health (1989c) *Working for Patients: Funding and Contracts for Hospital Services* (Working Paper 2). London: HMSO.

Department of Health (1989d) *Caring for People*. London: HMSO.

Department of Health (1990) *Health and Personal Social Services Statistics for England*, 1990. London. HMSO.

Department of Health (1992) *Healthy Alliances*. London: HMSO.

Dingwall, R., Rafferty, A. and Webster, C. (1988) *An Introduction to the Social History of Nursing*. London: Routledge.

Dixon, J. and Glennerster, H. (1995) What do we know about fundholding in general practice?, *British Medical Journal*, 311: 727–730.

Donaldson, L. (1995) The listening blank, *Health Service Journal*, 25 September: 22–24.

Dore, R. (1983) Goodwill and the spirit of market capitalism, *British Journal of Sociology*, 34(4): 459–82.

Duggan, M. (1995) *Primary Health Care*. London: Institute for Public Policy Research.

Dunleavy, P. (1981) 'Professions and policy change', *Public Administration Bulletin*, 36: 3–16.

Exworthy, M. (1994) The contest for control in community health services, *Policy and Politics*, 22(1): 17–29.

Ferlie, E. (1994) The evolution of quasi-markets in the NHS, in W. Bartlett *et al.* (eds) *Quasi-Markets in the Welfare State*. Bristol: School for Advanced Urban Studies.

Ferlie, E., Cairncross, L. and Pettigrew, M. (1993) Understanding internal markets in the NHS, in I. Tilley (ed.) *Managing the Internal Market*. London: Paul Chapman.

Fitzpatrick, R. (1994) Health needs assessment, chronic illness and the social sciences, in J. Popay and G. Williams (eds) *Researching the People's Health*. London: Routledge.

Flynn, R. (1992a) *Structures of Control in Health Management*. London: Routledge.

Flynn, R. (1992b) Managed markets – producers and consumers in the NHS, in R. Burrows and C. Marsh (eds.) *Consumption and Class*. London: Macmillan.

Fox, A. (1974) *Beyond Contract*. London: Faber and Faber.

Frances, J., Levacic, R., Mitchell, J. and Thompson, G. (1991) Introduction, in *Markets, Hierarchies and Networks*. London: Sage.

Freemantle, N., Watt, I. and Mason, J. (1993) Developments in the purchasing process in the NHS. *Public Administration*, 71, Winter: 535–48.

Gaster, L. (1995) *Quality in Public Services*. Buckingham: Open University Press.

Giddens, A. (1991) *Consequences of Modernity*. Cambridge: Polity Press.

Glennerster, H., Matsaganis, M. and Owens, P. (1992) *A Foothold for Fundholding*. London: King's Fund Institute.

Glennerster, H., Matasaganis, M., Owens, P. and Hancock, S. (1994) *Implementing GP Fundholding*. Buckingham: Open University Press.

Goss, S., Isaacs, J., Little, D., and Stratford, M. (1993) The champions, *Health Service Journal*, July: 34–5.

Granovetter, M. (1985) Economic action and social structure – the problem of embeddedness, *American Journal of Sociology*, 91(3), 481–510.

Granovetter, M. (1992) Economic institutions as social constructions, *Acta Sociologica*, 35(3): 3–11.

Gray, A. and Jenkins, W. (1993) Markets, managers and the public service, in P. Taylor-Gooby and R. Lawson, *Markets and Managers*. Buckingham Open University Press.

Ham, C. (1994a) *Management and Competition in the New NHS*. Oxford: Radcliffe Medical Press.

Ham, C. (1994b) Reforming health services, *Social Policy and Administration*, 28(4): 293–8.

Hammersley, M. (1990) *Reading Ethnographic Research*. London: Longman.

Hammersley, M. and Atkinson, P. (1983) *Ethnography: Principles in Practice*. London: Tavistock.

Hancock, C. (1995) Invest in a long-term relationship, *Health Services Journal*, 2 March: 21.

Harden, I. (1992) *The Contracting State*. Buckingham: Open University Press.

Hardy, B., Wistow, G. and Rhodes, R. A. W. (1990) Policy networks and the implementation of community care policy, *Journal of Social Policy*, 19(2): 141–68.

Harrison, A. (1993) *From Hierarchy to Contract*. Hermitage: Policy Journals and Transaction Books.

Harrison, S. and Wistow, G. (1992) The purchaser–provider split in English health care, *Policy and Politics*, 20(2): 123–130.

Harrison, S., Hunter, D., Johnston, I. and Wistow, G. (1989) *Competing for Health*. Leeds: Nuffield Institute for Health Service Studies.

Harrison, S., Hunter, D. and Pollitt, C. (1990) *The Dynamics of British Health Policy*. London: Unwin Hyman.

Health and Personal Social Services Statistics for England 1995, London: HMSO, Government Statistical Office.

Heydebrand, W. V. (1989) New organizational forms, *Work and Occupations*, 16(3): 323–57.

Hjern, B. and Porter, D. (1981) Implementation structures, *Organization Studies*, 2/3: 211–27.

Hudson, B. (1995) Joint commissioning, *Policy and Politics*, 23(3): 233–49.

Hugman, R. (1995) Contested territory and community services, in K. Soothill, L. Mackay and C. Webb (eds) *Interprofessional Relations in Health Care*. London: Edward Arnold.

Hunter, D. (1994) From tribalism to corporatism: the managerial challenge to medical dominance, in J. Gabe, D. Kelleher and G. Williams (eds) *Challenging Medicine*. London: Routledge.

Jackson, P. M. (1994) The new public sector management, in P. Jackson and C. Marsh (eds) *Privatisation and Regulation*. Harlow: Longman.

Jost, T., Hughes, D., McHale, J. and Griffith, L. (1995) The British health care reforms, the American health care revolution and purchaser–provider contracts, *Journal of Health Politics, Policy and Law*, 20(4): 886–908.

Kerrison, S. (1993) Contracting and the quality of medical care, in I. Tilley (ed.) *Managing the Internal Market*. Liverpool: Paul Chapman.

Key, P., Deardon, B. and Lund, B. (1994) Perspectives on purchasing: private lessons, *Health Services Journal*, 27 January: 27–9.

Knapp, M., Wistow, G., Forder, J. and Hardy, B. (1994) Markets for social care, in W. Bartlett, C. Propper, D. Wilson and J. Le Grand (eds) *Quasi-Markets in the Welfare State*. Bristol: School for Advanced Urban Studies.

Knights, D., Murray, F. and Willmott, H. (1993) Networking as knowledge work, *Journal of Management Studies*, 30(6): 975–95.

Larson, A. (1992) Network dyads in entrepreneurial settings, *Administrative Science Quarterly*, 37: 76–104.

Le Grand, J. (1990) Quasi-markets and social policy, *Studies in Decentralisation and Quasi-Markets 1*. Bristol: School for Advanced Urban Studies.

Le Grand, J. (1994) Evaluating the NHS reforms, in R. Robinson and J. Le Grand (eds) *Evaluating the NHS Reforms*. Hermitage: Policy Journals.

Levacic, R. (1993) Markets as coordinative devices, in R. Maidment and G. Thompson (eds) *Managing the UK*. London: Sage.

Lightfoot, J. (1994) The accountable professional in the NHS, in A. Harrison (ed.) *Health Care UK 1993–4*. London: King's Fund Institute.

Lightfoot, J., Baldwin, S. and Wright, K. (1992) *Nursing by Numbers*. University of York: Social Policy Research Unit.

Lightfoot, J., Baldwin, S. and Wright, K. (undated) *Community Nursing Study: report on a study of establishment setting*, DH 947.6.92. University of York: Social Policy Research Unit.

Lincoln, J. R. (1990) Japanese organization and organization theory, *Research in Organizational Behavior*, 12, 255–94.

Long, A. (1994) Assessing health and social outcomes, in J. Popay and G. Williams (eds) *Researching the People's Health*. London: Routledge.

Luhmann, N. (1979) *Trust and Power*. Chichester: John Wiley.

Luhmann, N. (1988) Familiarity, confidence, trust, in D. Gambetta (ed.) *Trust*. Oxford: Blackwell.

Lupton, C. and Taylor, P. (1995) Coming in from the cold, *Health Service Journal*, March: 22–24.

Mackerrel, D. (1993) Contract pricing, in I. Tilley (ed.) *Managing the Internal Market*. Liverpool: Paul Chapman.

Mackintosh, M. (1993) Economic behaviour and the contracting outcome under the NHS reforms, *Accounting, Auditing and Accountability Journal*, (6)3: 133–55.

Maheswaran, S. and Appleby, J. (1992) Building quality standards into contracts, *Health Direct*, September: 6.

Maynard, A. (1993) Creating competition in the NHS, in I. Tilley (ed.) *Managing the Internal Market*. Liverpool: Paul Chapman.

Means, R., Hoyes, L., Lart, R., and Taylor, M. (1994) Quasi-markets and social care: towards user empowerment?, in W. Bartlett, C. Propper, D. Wilson and J. Le Grand (eds) *Quasi-markets in the Welfare State*. Bristol: School for Advanced Urban Studies.

Medical Practitioners Union (1992) *The Future of Primary Care*. London: Medical World Supplement.

Morgan, G. (1990) *Organisations and Society*. Macmillan: London.

Morris, J. (1994) *The Shape of Things to Come? User-led Social Services*, Social Services Policy Forum paper 3. London: National Institute for Social Work.

National Association of Health Authorities and Trusts (1994) *Developing Contracting*. NAHAT discussion paper 15. Birmingham: NAHAT.

National Audit Office (1994) *General Practitioner Fundholding in England*. London: HMSO.

National Audit Office (1995) *Contracting for Acute Health Care in England*. Report by the Comptroller and Auditor General. London: HMSO.

National Consumer Council (1992) *Involving the Community: Guidelines for Health Service Managers*. London: NCC.

NHS Executive (1994a) *Purchasing for Health: Involving Local People*. Leeds: NHSE.

NHS Executive (1994b) EL(94) 79. *Developing NHS Purchasing and GP Fundholding*. Leeds: NHSE.

NHS Executive (1994c) *1995–6 Contracting Review: Handbook* EL(94)88. Leeds: NHSE.

NHS Executive (1995) *Priorities and Planning Guidance for the NHS 1996–7*. Leeds: NHSE.

NHS Executive (1996) Personal communication, 14 February 1996. Leeds: Department of Health, Leeds.

NHS Management Executive (1990a) *Working for Patients – NHS Trusts: a Working Guide.* London: HMSO.

NHS Management Executive (1990b) *Working for Patients: Contracts for Health Services – Operating Contracts*. London: NHSME.

NHS Management Executive (1990d) *Nursing in the Community*. London: NHSME.

NHS Management Executive (1991) *Assessing Health Care Needs*. London: NHSME.

NHS Management Executive (1992) *Local Voices*. Leeds: NHSME.

NHS Management Executive, Information Management Group (1993a) *Developing Information Systems for Purchasers. Thinking Ahead.* Leeds: DISP/NHSME.

NHS Management Executive, Information Management Group (1993b) *Community Information Systems for Providers. Describing Community Care.* Leeds: CISP/NHSME.

NHS Management Executive, Information Management Group (1993c) *Community Information System for Providers. Improving Contracting Data.* Leeds: CISP/NHSME.

NHS Management Executive (1993d) *Costing for Contracting*, EL(93)26. Leeds: NHSME.

NHS Management Executive (1994) *The Operation of the NHS Internal Market*, HSG(94)55. Leeds: NHSME.

O'Keefe, E., Ottewill, R. and Wall, A. (1992) *Community Health: Issues in Management.* Sunderland, Tyne and Wear: Business Education Publishers Limited.

Ottewill, R. and Wall, A. (1990) *The Growth and Development of the Community Health Services*. Sunderland, Tyne and Wear: Business Education Publishers Limited.

Ouchi, W. (1991) Markets, bureaucracies and clans, in G. Thompson *et al. Markets, Hierarchies and Networks*. London: Sage.

Øvretveit, J. (1992) *Health Service Quality*. Edinburgh: Blackwell Scientific Publications.

Øvretveit, J. (1993) *Coordinating Community Care*. Buckingham: Open University Press.

Øvretveit, J. (1995) *Purchasing for Health*. Buckingham: Open University Press.

Paton, C. (1992) *Competition and Planning in the NHS – The Danger of Unplanned Markets*, London: Chapman and Hall.

Perrow, C. (1981) Markets, hierarchies and hegemony, in A. van de Ven and W. Joyce (eds) *Perspectives on Organization Design and Behavior*. New York: John Wiley.

Pettigrew, A. (1990) Longitudinal field research on change, *Organization Science*, 1(3): 267–92.

Pickard, S., Williams, G. and Flynn, R. (1995) 'Local voices in an internal market', *Social Policy and Administration*, 29(2): 135–49.

Pickin, C. and St. Leger, S. (1993) *Assessing Health Need Using the Life Cycle Framework*. Buckingham: Open University Press.

Pilgrim, D. and Rogers, A. (1993) *Experiencing Psychiatry: Users' Views of Services*. London: Macmillan.

Plamping, D. and Delamothe, T. (1991) The Citizen's Charter and the NHS, *British Medical Journal*, 303 (6796): 203–4.

Pollitt, C. (1990) *Managerialism and the Public Services*. Oxford: Blackwell.

Pollitt, C., Harrison, S., Hunter, D.J. and Marnoch, G. (1990) No hiding place, *Journal of Social Policy*, 19(2): 169–90.

Pollock, A. and Majeed, F. (1991) Community oriented primary care, *British Medical Journal*, 310: 481–2.

Popay, J. and Williams, G. (1993) Sociological approaches to collecting information on health needs, in C. Pickin and S. St Leger, *Assessing Health Need in the Life Cycle Framework*. Buckingham: Open University Press.

Popay, J. and Williams, G. (eds) (1994a) *Researching the People's Health*. London: Routledge.

Popay, J. and Williams, G. H. (1994b) Local voices in the NHS: needs, effectiveness and sufficiency, in A. Oakley and S. Williams (eds) *The Politics of the Welfare State*. London: Routledge.

Potter, J. (1988) Consumerism and the public sector, *Public Administration*, 66(2):149–64.

Powell, W. (1991) Neither market nor hierarchy: network forms of organisation, in G. Thompson *et al.* (eds) *Markets, Hierarchies and Networks*. London: Sage.

Propper, C. (1993) Quasi-markets. Contracts and quality in health and social care, in J. Le Grand and W. Bartlett (eds) *Quasi-Markets and Social Policy*. London: Macmillan.

Propper, C., Bartlett, W. and Wilson, D. (1994) Introduction, in W. Bartlett *et al.* (eds) *Quasi-Markets in the Welfare State*. Bristol: School for Advanced Urban Studies.

Ranade, W. (1992) *Perspectives on the Market*. NAHAT project paper 6. Birmingham: National Association of Health Authorities and Trusts.

Ranade, W. (1994) *A Future for the NHS?* London: Longman.

Rea, D. (1995) Unhealthy competition, *Policy and Politics*, 23(2): 141–55.

Reed, M. (1992) *The Sociology of Organizations*. Hemel Hempstead: Harvester Wheatsheaf.

Reid, B. (1995) Interorganisational networks and the delivery of local housing services, *Housing Studies*, 10(2): 133–49.

Reve, T. (1990) The firm as a nexus of internal and external contracts, in M. Aoki, B. Gustaffson and O. Williamson (eds) *The Firm as a Nexus of Treaties*. London: Sage.

Ring, P. S. and Van Den Ven, A. H. (1992) Structuring cooperative relations between organizations, *Strategic Management Journal*, 13: 483–98.

Robin, N. (1992) Beware GPs bearing wallets, *Health Visitor*, 65: 3.

Robinson, R. (1993) Checks and balances, *Health Service Journal*. 2 September: 30–1.

Robinson, R. (1994) Markets and health care, in P. Jackson and C. Price (eds) *Privatisation and Regulation*. Harlow: Longman.

Rosen, M. (1991) Coming to terms with the field – understanding and doing organizational ethnography, *Journal of Management Studies*, 28(1): 1–24.

Saltman, R. and von Otter, C. (1992) *Planned Markets and Public Competition*. Milton Keynes: Open University Press.

Scott, J. (1991) *Social Network Analysis*. London: Sage.

Shackley, P. and Ryan, M. (1994) What is the role of the consumer in health care?, *Journal of Social Policy*, 23(4): 517–41.

Shapiro, J. (1994) A time to share, *Health Service Journal*, 3 November: 24–5.

Small, N. (1989) *Politics and Planning in the National Health Service*. Milton Keynes: Open University Press.

Smith, P. (1994) The Nature of Contracts in the British National Health Service: Paper presented at the Conference of the Association for Research on Nonprofit Organizations and Voluntary Action, 10–22 October, Berkeley, California.

Smith P., Mackintosh M. and Towers, B. (1993) Implications of the new NHS contracting system for the district nursing service, *Journal of Interprofessional Care*, 7(2): 115–24.

Spurgeon, P. (1993) Regulation or free market for the NHS?, in I. Tilley, (ed.) *Managing the Internal Market*. Liverpool: Paul Chapman.

Spurgeon P. and Smith, P. (1995) Living with Contracts: Paper presented at the Conference on NHS Reforms, 12 May, University of Swansea.

Stockford, D. (1993) Perspectives on purchasing, *Health Services Journal*, 9 December: 20–3.

Strong, P. and Robinson, J. (1990) *The NHS Under New Management*. Milton Keynes: Open University Press.

Swedberg, R. and Granovetter, M. (1992) Introduction, in M. Granovetter and R. Swedberg (eds) *The Sociology of Economic Life*. Boulder and Oxford: Westview Press.

Taylor, D. (1991) *Developing Primary Care: Opportunities for the 1990s*. London: King's Fund Institute.

Taylor-Gooby, P. and Lawson, M. (1993) Where we go from here, in P. Taylor-Gooby and R. Lawson, *Markets and Managers*. Buckingham: Open University Press.

Thompson, G. (1993) Network coordination, in R. Maidment and G. Thompson (eds) *Managing the UK*. London: Sage.

Thompson, P. (1993) Postmodernism – fatal distraction, in J. Hassard and M. Parker (eds) *Postmodernism and Organizations*. London: Sage.

Thorelli, H. B. (1990) Networks – between markets and hierarchies, in D. Ford (ed.) *Understanding Business Markets*. London: Academic Press.

Traynor, M. (1995) *A Study of Three NHS Trusts: the Managers' Account*. Report IV. London: Royal College of Nursing.

Traynor, M. and Wade, B. (1994) *The Morale of Nurses working in the community*. Report III. London: Royal College of Nursing.

Turk, J. (1983) Power, efficiency and institutions, in A. Francis, J. Turk and P. Willman (eds) *Power, Efficiency and Institutions*. London: Heinemann Educational.

Twigg, J. and Atkin, K. (1994) *Carers Perceived*. Buckingham: Open University Press.

Walsh, K. (1995) *Public Services and Market Mechanisms*. Basingstoke: Macmillan.

Williams, S., Calnan, M., Cant, S. and Coyle, J. (1993) All change in the NHS?, *Sociology of Health and Illness*, 15(1): 43–67.

Williamson, O.E. (1983) *Markets and Hierarchies*. New York: Free Press.

Williamson, O.E. (1985) *The Economic Institutions of Capitalism*. New York: Free Press.

Williamson, O.E. (1991) Comparative economic organization, *Administrative Science Quarterly*, 36: 269–96.

Williamson, O. E. and Ouchi, W. (1983) The markets and hierarchies programme of research, in A. Francis, J. Turk and P. Willman (eds) *Power, Efficiency and Institutions*. London: Heinemann Educational.

Wistow, G., Knapp, M., Hardy, B. and Allen, C. (1994) *Social Care in a Mixed Economy*. Buckingham: Open University Press.

Index

SOCIAL CARE IN A MIXED ECONOMY

Gerald Wistow, Martin Knapp, Brian Hardy and Caroline Allen

This book describes the mixed economy of community care in England and analyses the efforts and activities of local authorities to promote and develop it. It is based on national documentary and statistical evidence and on more detailed research with twenty-four local authorities; and includes a case study on the transfer of residential homes to the independent sector.

The roles of social services departments have been progressively redefined to emphasize responsibility for creating and managing a mixed economy. This entails a major cultural shift for departments which may be summarized as involving moves from providing to enabling, and from administration to management. It also implies the need for new skills and structures. *Social Care in a Mixed Economy* traces the historical changes; the local interpretations of central government policy; how authorities actually have been developing mixed economies; the main opportunities or incentives for promoting a mixed economy; and the main obstacles to its development.

Contents
Introduction: historical and policy context – Community care: markets and enabling – The mixed economy in 1991 – Local responses to the legislation and guidance – Building a mixed economy – Social care is different – Residential care home transfers – Conclusions – Appendix – References – Name index – Subject index.

176pp   0 335 19043 X (Paperback)   0 335 19044 8 (Hardback)

COORDINATING COMMUNITY CARE
MULTIDISCIPLINARY TEAMS AND CARE MANAGEMENT

John Øvretveit

This book is about how people from different professions and agencies work together to meet the health and social needs of people in a community. It is about making the most of different skills to meet people's needs, and creating satisfying and supportive working groups. It is about the details of making community care a reality.

The effectiveness and quality of care a person receives depends on getting the right professionals and services, and also on the support given to the person's carers. Services must be coordinated if the person is to benefit, but coordination is more difficult with the increasing change, variety and complexity of health and social services in the 1990s. This book challenges the assumptions that services are best coordinated by multi-professional and multi-agency teams, and that community care teams are broadly similar. It demonstrates when a team is needed and how to overcome differences between professions, and between agency policies and philosophies.

Drawing on ten years of consultancy research with a variety of teams and services, the author gives practical guidance for managers and practitioners about how to set up and improve coordination and teamwork. The book combines practical concerns with theoretical depth drawing on organization and management theory, psychology, psycho-analysis, sociology, economics and government studies.

Contents
Introduction – Needs and organization – Markets, bureaucracy and association – Types of team – Client pathways and team resource management – Team members' roles – Team leadership – Decisions and conflict in teams – Communications and co-service – Coordinating community health and social care – Appendices – Glossary – References and bibliography – Index.

240pp   0 335 19047 2 (Paperback)

IMPLEMENTING COMMUNITY CARE

Nigel Malin (ed.)

This introductory text provides a unique overview of the implementation of community care policy and the process of managing changes in the field. The central thesis is an expansion of the theme of integrating policy and professional practice in order to assess the requirements for providing models of care based upon a user and care management perspective. The book analyses the impact of changes for community nurses, social workers, those employed in residential and home-based care and discusses anticipated new roles and functions. Its examination of changes in policy and planning both at national and local level makes it a valuable sourcebook for health care, social work practitioners and planners, but the volume is designed for use by students and professionals alike. The emphasis throughout is on the design and delivery of services and providing an overview of research findings, particularly in relation to measuring service effectiveness.

Contents
Preface – Section 1: The policy context – Development of community care – Management and finance – Community care planning – Care management – Section 2: Staff and users – The caring professions – The family and informal care – Measuring service quality – The consumer role – Section 3: Models for care – Residential services – Day services – Domiciliary services – Index.

Contributors
Andy Alaszewski, Michael Beazley, John Brown, David Challis, Brian Hardy, Bob Hudson, Aileen McIntosh, Steve McNally, Nigel Malin, Jill Manthorpe, Jim Monarch, John Rose, Len Spriggs, Gerald Wistow, Wai-Ling Wun.

224pp   0 335 15738 6 (Paperback)